Color Atlas and Synopsis of Sexually Transmitted Diseases

W9-CPE-829

Color Atlas and Synopsis of Sexually Transmitted Diseases

H. Hunter Handsfield, M.D.

Professor of Medicine
University of Washington School of Medicine
Director, STD Control Program
Seattle–King County Department of Public Health
Seattle, Washington

McGRAW-HILL, INC.
Health Professions Division
New York   St. Louis   San Francisco   Auckland
Bogotá   Caracas   Lisbon   London   Madrid   Mexico
Milan   Montreal   New Delhi   Paris   San Juan
Singapore   Sydney   Tokyo   Toronto

Color Atlas and Synopsis of Sexually Transmitted Diseases

1 2 3 4 5 6 7 8 9 0 KGS KGS 9 8 7 6 5 4 3 2 1

This book was set in Garamond by Arcata Graphics/Kingsport. The editors
were J. Dereck Jeffers and Lester A. Sheinis. The production supervisor was
Richard Ruzycka. The cover was designed by NSG Design. Arcata
Graphics/Kingsport was printer and binder.

ISBN 0-07-026006-0

Library of Congress Cataloging-in-Publication Data

Handsfield. H. Hunter.
    Color atlas and synopsis of sexually transmitted diseases/H.
Hunter Handsfield.
      p.   cm.
    Includes bibliographical references and index.
    ISBN 0-07-026006-0
    1. Sexually transmitted diseases—Atlases.   2. Sexually
transmitted diseases—Outlines, syllabi, etc.   I. Title.
    [DNLM: 1. Sexually Transmitted Diseases—atlases.   2. Sexually
Transmitted Diseases—outlines.   WC   17   H236c]
    RC200.H36   1992
    616.95′1—dc20
    DNLM/DLC
    for Library of Congress   91–25390
                                                                         CIP

This book is dedicated with love and respect
to my father,
Hugh W. Handsfield,
for 40 years an editor and editor-in-chief of the
McGraw-Hill College Division.
He always wanted a
McGraw-Hill author in the family.

Contents

Preface

Until 45 years ago, sexually transmitted diseases were part of the medical mainstream. Gonorrhea, syphilis, and their complications were common throughout society, and most physicians were prepared to diagnose patients and to manage or refer them to specialists. Skilled care was available at major medical centers and teaching hospitals, where dermatovenereology clinics often were among the largest clinical programs. Many medical students and residents received substantial training in these clinics. Then penicillin became available. Treatment no longer required highly trained specialists, the number of patients with recognized complications declined, municipal and state health departments assumed increasing responsibility for diagnosis and treatment, and STD care gravitated away from the medical centers. This trend was abetted by the belief that STDs soon would be eradicated and perhaps by the willingness of some physicians to relinquish responsibility for "that kind" of patient. Probably for the same reasons, health departments saw little need to provide the sophisticated, aesthetic settings that might have helped to attract excellent physicians and enthusiastic trainees. Venereology became a backwater field.

Thus, a generation and a half of physicians and other health care providers—the large majority of those now in practice—had no role models and received little or no training in STDs. As a result, the medical profession was totally unprepared for three developments. First, the sexual revolution and related social changes placed most people at risk for STD for much of their lives. STDs never were limited to "that kind" of patient, but now it became obvious. Second, advances in microbiology, immunology, and epidemiology defined a panoply of previously unrecognized STDs; most were difficult to recognize, hard or impossible to treat, and yet caused serious, long-lasting sequelae. In addition, the sexual revolution led to a resurgence of the old STDs. The third development was the explosive appearance of AIDS, the most devastating STD of all time.

Even now, very little time is devoted to educating health sciences students about STDs other than AIDS. Most physicians complete five to ten years of training with no more than four hours of lectures on the subject and diagnose or knowingly manage few if any patients with STDs before entering practice. This atlas and synopsis is written for such clinicians and health sciences students, who find themselves confronted with patients with STD or at risk and need an easy-to-use aid to diagnosis and management. On the way to my present appointment, I spent two years in solo, private practice and can certify that all the clinical and diagnostic procedures described in this book are well within the capability of the basically trained clinician. Most of the necessary laboratory tests now are readily available at reasonable cost.

The case histories presented in this book are real, but some are composites of more than one patient. For some cases that occurred several years ago, the treatment described or tests performed were updated to conform with current recommendations. The majority of the photographs were taken of the patients described, but some photos—especially those provided by colleagues—lacked clinical information and were matched with patients with complete histories. In response to a common question, in all photographs the ungloved hands are the patients'.

As for most books, this work would not have been possible without the generous help of many colleagues. Drs. Larry Corey, Ann Collier, Julie McElrath, King Holmes, Phil Kirby, Sheila Lukehart, Walter Stamm, Bob Willkens, Bob Wood, Pål Wølner-Hanssen, and Fred Bushnell reviewed chapters and gave helpful advice. The staff of the Seattle–King County Department of Public Health STD Clinic at Harborview Medical Center referred patients for photography and were supportive friends; they truly make my job fun. Several of the photographs were taken by Roger Hartley of Pan Enterprises. Others were taken by the author, and some were kindly provided by various colleagues; these are credited. Oran Walker prepared the manuscript and ably provided other secretarial services. J. Dereck Jeffers and Lester A. Sheinis, my editors, were frustrated and often bemused by my tardiness but remained tactful in their prodding; I thoroughly enjoyed working with them.

Finally, I thank Patricia McInturff, Director of the Regional Services Division of the Seattle–King County Department of Public Health. As my supervisor, she permitted the necessary time from my other duties; as my wife, she provided encouragement despite the time the project took from our personal life.

Abbreviations

AIDS	Acquired immunodeficiency syndrome	**IM**	Intramuscular
BID	Twice daily	**IV**	Intravenous
BV	Bacterial vaginosis	**LGV**	Lymphogranuloma venereum
CDC	Centers for Disease Control, U.S. Public Health Service	**MHA-TP**	Microhemagglutination assay for *Treponema pallidum*
CMV	Cytomegalovirus	**MPC**	Mucopurulent cervicitis
EIA	Enzyme immunoassay	**NGU**	Nongonococcal urethritis
ELISA	Enzyme-linked immunosorbent assay	**PID**	Pelvic inflammatory disease
		PMN	Polymorphonuclear leukocyte
ESR	Erythrocyte sedimentation rate	**PO**	Per os (orally)
FTA-ABS	Fluorescent treponemal antibody-absorbed test	**QID**	Four times daily
		RPR	Rapid plasma reagin test
HBV	Hepatitis B virus	**STD**	Sexually transmitted disease
HIV	Human immunodeficiency virus	**TID**	Three times daily
HPV	Human papillomavirus	**VDRL**	Venereal Disease Research Laboratory test
HSV	Herpes simplex virus		
ICGND	Intracellular gram-negative diplococci		

Color Atlas and Synopsis of Sexually Transmitted Diseases

Overview of Sexually Transmitted Diseases

Chapter 1 Clinical Approach to Patients with STDs

INTRODUCTION

In few areas of infectious diseases have changes in the epidemiology and our understanding of clinical manifestations been as profound as in the field of sexually transmitted diseases (STDs) during the past two decades. Despite the predictions of the early antibiotic era, bacterial STDs remain epidemic, perhaps the best example of the influence that demographic, social, and behavioral factors can have on infectious diseases in the face of effective treatment and other preventive measures. In addition, the perceived spectrum of STD has broadened greatly through recognition of several "new" pathogens, syndromes, and complications.

Prevention and control of STD are largely women's health care issues. Many STDs appear to be transmitted more efficiently from men to women than the reverse, probably because the vagina serves as a reservoir that prolongs exposure to infectious secretions. Women are more likely than men to have asymptomatic infections or minor, nonspecific symptoms, resulting in delayed diagnosis. The diagnosis of STD is more difficult in women, because the clinical findings are less specific and several microbiologic tests are less sensitive than in men. Finally, women and their children are at greater risk than men for long-lasting or permanent sequelae.

Because of the sexual revolution and related societal changes, the majority of Americans now are at substantial risk for STD for large segments of their lives, and late complications continue to occur for years after persons at risk adopt lower risk lifestyles. Clinicians who formerly diagnosed and treated few cases now regularly provide care to patients with STD or at risk. As for all medical conditions, the first step in treatment, prevention, and control is clinical recognition and diagnosis, and these are the focus of this synopsis and atlas. This chapter presents an overview of the clinical approach to STD diagnosis and management, laying groundwork for the chapters to come.

CLASSIFICATION OF STD

STDs can be classified traditionally, according to the causative pathogenic organisms (Table 1-1). However, many STD syndromes are caused by more than one STD pathogen, and in some cases nonsexually transmitted agents contribute to pathogenesis. Table 1-2 shows the major STD clinical syndromes and complications, listed in the approximate order of their importance to human health. (Note that the first half of the list is dominated by syndromes that predominantly affect women and children.) Both the etiologic and syndromic organizations are used in this book.

Table 1-1
Sexually Transmitted Pathogens

BACTERIA	VIRUSES
Neisseria gonorrhoeae	Human immunodeficiency virus (types 1 and 2)
Trepomena pallidum	Herpes simplex virus (types 1 and 2)
Chlamydia trachomatis	Human papillomavirus (many types)
Haemophilis ducreyi	Hepatitis viruses A, B, C, and D
Calymmatobacterium granulomatis	Cytomegalovirus
Ureaplasma urealyticum	Epstein-Barr virus
Mycoplasma hominis	Molluscum contagiosum virus
Mycoplasma genitalium	Enteric viruses
Gardnerella vaginalis	
Salmonella sp.	
Shigella sp.	
Campylobacter sp.	
Streptococcus group B	
Mobiluncus sp.	

PROTOZOA	ECTOPARASITES
Trichomonas vaginalis	*Phthirus pubis* (pubic louse)
Entamoeba histolytica	*Sarcoptes scabiei* (scabies mite)
Giardia lamblia	
Other enteric protozoa	

POPULATIONS AT RISK

Recognition of social and demographic markers for STD is the first step in assessing risk and in clinical management. Population subgroups with the frequencies of new sexual partnerships and other poorly understood behavioral factors required to sustain an STD in the community are defined as core transmitters. Other persons acquire STD by sexual contact with core group members, but infection is not indefinitely propagated outside the core. The core populations for gonorrhea and syphilis consist primarily of young, ethnic minority persons of low socioeconomic level, with high rates of illicit drug use and prostitution, often residing within circumscribed high-prevalence geographic areas. The core group is substantially broader for chlamydial infection than for gonorrhea, partly because coordinated control measures such as widespread screening are not undertaken in most communities. For genital herpes, human papillomavirus infection, and other persistent viral STDs, the "core" may encompass most of the population.

Table 1-2
Major STD Clinical Syndromes and Complications

1. Acquired immunodeficiency syndrome and related conditions
2. Pelvic inflammatory disease
3. Female infertility and ectopic pregnancy
4. Fetal and neonatal infections: conjunctivitis, pneumonia, pharyngeal infection, encephalitis, cognitive impairment, deformities, deafness, immunodeficiency, death
5. Complications of pregnancy and delivery: spontaneous abortion, premature labor, premature rupture of fetal membranes, chorioamnionitis, postpartum endometritis
6. Neoplasia: cervical dysplasia and carcinoma, Kaposi's sarcoma, hepatocellular carcinoma, squamous cell carcinomas of anus, vulva, and penis
7. Human papillomavirus infection and genital warts
8. Genital ulcer–inguinal lymphadenopathy syndromes
9. Lower genital tract infection in women: cervicitis, urethritis, vaginal infection
10. Viral hepatitis and cirrhosis
11. Urethritis in men
12. Late syphilis
13. Epididymitis
14. Gastrointestinal infections: proctitis, enteritis, colitis
15. Acute arthritis
16. Mononucleosis syndrome
17. Molluscum contagiosum
18. Ectoparasite infestation (scabies, pubic lice)

MEDICAL AND SEXUAL HISTORY

Assessment of risk requires an accurate social and sexual history, including appraisal of factors that influence sexuality, such as substance abuse. Broaching the subject is often daunting, because of personal anxieties and perceptions about these issues, because the clinician may lack specific training, and, perhaps most important, because the process is viewed as requiring more time than a busy practice may allow. However, a forthright and sensitive approach usually results in accurate data and usually need not take more than two or three minutes. The medical history also can be succinct yet complete. The Appendix presents the elements of the medical and sexual history obtained routinely at the author's STD clinic.

PHYSICAL EXAMINATION

The physical examination of patients with STD or at risk is straightforward (see Appendix). All patients require inspection of the entire skin surface, although this may be cursory in patients without cutaneous symptoms and in whom syphilis is unlikely. In our STD clinic, at a minimum we carefully inspect all skin surfaces that are uncovered or are normally exposed during the genital examination, including the face, head, hands, lower arms, lower trunk, pubic area, and thighs. The mouth and throat are examined and the neck, supra-clavicular fossae, axillae, and inguinal areas are palpated for lymphadenopathy.

In men, the genitals and the pubic and inguinal regions are carefully inspected; the foreskin is retracted and the penis is palpated, including "milking" the urethra from the urethral bulb distally to express discharge; and the scrotum is palpated for masses, tenderness, and other abnormalities. For homosexually active men, the anus and perineum are carefully inspected. The examination of women includes inspection of the pubic area, the external genitals, perineum and anus, speculum examination of the vaginal mucosa and cervix, and a bimanual pelvic examination. For men or women with symptoms suggestive of proctitis or proctocolitis, the rectal mucosa is examined through an anoscope.

LABORATORY DIAGNOSIS

Although many STDs can be suspected or diagnosed presumptively on clinical grounds, numerous readily available laboratory tests are underutilized. Clinicians treating patients with STD should have immediate access to serologic tests for human immunodeficiency virus (HIV) infection and syphilis, culture for *Neisseria gonorrhoeae,* culture or antigen-detection tests for *Chlamydia trachomatis* and herpes simplex virus (HSV), microscopy for examination of Gram-stained smears and wet mounts of vaginal secretions, and cervical cytology. Clinicians who serve patients at high risk for syphilis should have access to dark-field microscopy and rapid serologic tests, such as the rapid plasma reagin card test.

- Most cases of gonorrhea should be confirmed by culture. The widespread occurrence of resistant gonococci now demands the availability of the organism for susceptibility testing in the event of treatment failure or recurrence.

- Most cases of chlamydial infection will not be detected or treated unless culture or antigen-detection tests for *C. trachomatis* are used liberally for screening and diagnosis.

- Classical cases of genital herpes can be diagnosed clinically. However, atypical presentations are common, and tests to detect HSV are indicated for all patients with genital ulcers, especially those not characteristic of herpes or syphilis.

- The most common lower genital tract infections in women—bacterial vaginosis, tricho-moniasis, candidiasis, and mucopurulent cervicitis—often are difficult to differentiate clinically and require microscopic or microbiologic tests for accurate diagnosis.

- Papanicolaou smears should be routinely obtained in women with STD or at risk, because they have the highest prevalences of premalignant dysplasia and overt malignancy.

- In settings in which syphilis is common, diagnosis and treatment before the patient leaves the office are important to prevent complications and to curtail transmission to other persons. This requires dark-field microscopy or immediate serologic testing.

SELECTION OF TREATMENT

Several factors influence the selection of treatment for patients with STD, in addition to the standard ones of activity of the drug against the infecting pathogen, potential toxicity, and cost.

- The likelihood of concurrent STDs should be considered. Because of the high rate of coexisting chlamydial infection or syphilis, treatment for gonorrhea should be effective against these infections.

- Single-dose treatment regimens are preferred when practical, especially for patients whose compliance is likely to be poor. Similarly, regimens with less frequent dosing are preferred (e.g., doxycycline BID instead of tetracycline QID). When multiple-dose regimens are used, careful counseling by the clinician can enhance adherence to treatment.

- The pharmacokinetic characteristics of an antibiotic and its differential efficacy at various anatomic sites of infection often affect selection of treatment. For example, benzathine penicillin therapy is effective for most cases of syphilis, but is unreliable if the central nervous system is infected. Similarly, some regimens that cure genital gonorrhea are less effective for pharyngeal infection.

- Convenience of administration, for both patient and clinician, may be a significant issue, especially in settings with rapid patient turnover (e.g., in STD clinics). As examples, single-dose oral therapy is easier than an IM injection, and some agents are easier to give by injection than others.

MANAGEMENT OF SEX PARTNERS

Management of the partner(s) is integral to treating patients with STD. Failure to examine and treat the partner often is tantamount to not treating the index case, who may be reinfected. Of course, notification also is important in limiting spread to other persons. The physician should take specific steps to examine the partners personally. For example, reproductive health clinics should be available to evaluate the partners of their female patients with STD, and health maintenance organizations should be available to partners of members. Alternatively, the clinician should assist in making a specific appointment for the partner elsewhere; vague advice that "your partner should be checked" is often unheeded.

It is unwise to give the patient medication for his or her partner. This practice often leads to incomplete treatment; other STDs that were not apparent in the index case may be missed; and the opportunity is lost to counsel the partner about sexual safety and to bring other sexual partners to treatment. Finally, there is significant medicolegal risk in treating a person who has not been personally examined. Nevertheless, such blind treatment may be warranted if the partner is remote from medical care or in other special circumstances.

COUNSELING

The clinician who treats a patient with STD should help the patient reduce his or her future risk of infection. Sexual safety should be addressed in all young people, using the same forthright but sensitive approach that works for the medical and sexual history. Sexual abstinence or maintenance of a permanent, mutually monogamous relationship should be emphasized, as should the use of condoms (preferably combined with spermicides) for all nonmonogamous sexual encounters that involve penile penetration into any orifice. In some populations, especially adolescents, monogamy may last only a few weeks, followed by a new monogamous relationship. The extremely high rates of STD in sexually active teenagers may be related more to such "serial monogamy" than to multiple simultaneous partnerships. Therefore, most unmarried persons <20 years old should be advised to use condoms for all sexual exposures, even in apparently committed relationships. Education and counseling also should address selectivity in choosing sexual partners, the recognition of symptoms of STD, and the links between STD and substance abuse. For most persons at risk, education and counseling based on pragmatic rationales are more readily accepted than advice justified on moral or religious grounds.

PARTNER NOTIFICATION

Notification and referral of the sexual partners of persons with STD is a traditional component of programs to prevent syphilis and gonorrhea, and it clearly has value for chlamydial infection. Partner referral in HIV infection and other viral STDs has been controversial. However, clinical intervention now is available (e.g., zidovudine therapy for some HIV-infected patients, vaccination to prevent hepatitis B), and persons who are aware that they are infected or have been exposed may be more likely to avoid infecting others.

In many areas, the local or state health department will assist in partner notification for some STDs, such as syphilis, HIV infection, and some cases of gonorrhea or pelvic inflammatory disease. For most infections, however, the practical extent of the clinician's involvement is to carefully counsel the patient to inform the partner and refer him or her for examination. The patient often needs the clinician's assistance in determining which contacts should be notified, depending on the specific infection and its usual incubation period, the date of onset, and related considerations. This process can be integrated with risk-reduction counseling.

SCREENING

Each sexually transmitted infection should be viewed as a "sentinel event" that reflects unprotected sexual activity, and clinical management should always include screening for other common STDs. For patients presenting for routine health care, the criteria for screening depend on the local disease prevalence, sensitivity and specificity of the screening test, the consequences of the infection for the patient's health, the potential for transmission to other partners, and the cost of testing. Screening of persons who are at risk but lack specific symptoms or signs of infection has a central role in the control of gonorrhea, syphilis, chlamydial infection, and HIV infection.

- Syphilis serology should be automatic in all patients at risk or who have any STD. Screening of all pregnant women is required in most states.
- Screening tests for *C. trachomatis* should be done at least yearly in most sexually active young women and whenever any other STD is diagnosed. Tests for chlamydial infection

also are productive in young men with other STDs and in some other settings, such as juvenile detention facilities or STD clinics.

- Testing for gonorrhea should be routine in all patients with another STD and in selected other persons, primarily those identified as belonging to core transmitter groups.
- Counseling about HIV prevention and serologic testing for HIV infection (with consent) should be routine for all patients with another STD or at risk, in addition to patients with other specific HIV risks, such as homosexually active men, IV drug users, and their sexual partners.

REPORTING

Documentation of STD morbidity is essential to control. Such data are necessary for the rational design of prevention programs, and resources can be directed to the core populations only if their occurrence, location, and demographic characteristics are known. Gonorrhea, syphilis, hepatitis B, and overt AIDS are universally reportable, and chlamydial infection now is reportable in most states. Some states also require reporting of all patients with HIV infection, first-episode genital herpes, and nongonococcal pelvic inflammatory disease. Clinicians should be familiar with local regulations and report all cases of designated STDs; failure to do so contributes to the continued spread of infection.

ADDITIONAL READING

Aral SO, Holmes KK: Sexually transmitted diseases in the AIDS era. *Scientific American* 264(2):62, 1991.

Berg AO: The primary care physician and sexually transmitted diseases control, in *Sexually Transmitted Diseases,* 2d ed, KK Holmes et al (eds). New York, McGraw-Hill, 1990, chap 93.

Brandt AM: *No Magic Bullet: A Social History of Venereal Disease in the United States since 1890,* 2d ed. New York, Oxford, 1989.

Cates W Jr: Epidemiology and control of sexually transmitted diseases: Strategic evolution. *Infect Dis Clin North Am* 1:1, 1987.

Centers for Disease Control: Sexually transmitted diseases treatment guidelines, 1989. *MMWR* 38(suppl 8), 1989.

Holmes KK et al (eds): *Sexually Transmitted Diseases,* 2d ed. New York, McGraw-Hill, 1990.

Bacterial Sexually Transmitted Diseases

Chapter 2   Gonorrhea

Gonorrhea is among the most common and widely recognized STDs throughout the world. *Neisseria gonorrhoeae,* a gram-negative diplococcus that in clinical material typically appears within neutrophils, primarily affects the mucosal surfaces of the urethra or endocervix and secondarily those of the rectum, pharynx, and conjunctivae. Ascending infection in women results in gonococcal pelvic inflammatory disease, the primary complication and a major cause of female infertility. Other complications include acute epididymitis, blindness resulting from corneal scarring, and bacteremic dissemination that results in a characteristic arthritis-dermatitis syndrome and rarely in bacterial endocarditis or meningitis. The spread of strains of *N. gonorrhoeae* with relative or absolute resistance to antibiotics has rendered the penicillins unsuitable for routine treatment of gonorrhea throughout the world.

EPIDEMIOLOGY

Incidence   Declining incidence in the United States in late 1980s; 692,000 cases reported (estimated 1.0–1.3 million total) in 1990, or 278 cases per 100,000 population (down from 468 per 100,000 in 1975); varies greatly between populations and geographic areas, with most cases occurring in urban, low socioeconomic populations

Prevalence   From 10–30 percent of patients in most urban STD clinics and many corrections facilities; 0.5–5 percent of women in family planning clinics; 0–2 percent of young, sexually active women in private physicians' offices

Transmission   Primarily by persons with asymptomatic or mildly symptomatic infection; most efficient by vaginal or anal intercourse, less so by orogenital exposure; efficient transmission to newborns during vaginal delivery

Age   All ages susceptible; >90 percent aged 15–34

Sex   Male:female ratio in United States currently 1.2:1, but highly variable

Race   In the United States, incidence is several times higher in black, Hispanic, and Native American than in white and Asian populations, but varies widely

Sexual Orientation   From 1970s to mid-1980s, homosexual and bisexual men had estimated incidence ≥10-fold higher than heterosexuals; currently rate similar to heterosexuals; occurs rarely, if ever, in exclusively homosexual women

Other Risk Markers   Unmarried, urban residence, lower educational and socioeconomic levels, illicit drug use, prostitution or sexual exposure to prostitutes, previous gonorrhea; increased risk in women who use no contraception or use nonbarrier methods; possible increased risk in women who use birth control pills for contraception (controversial)

HISTORY

Incubation Period   Typically 2–5 days for urethritis, 5–10 days for cervical infection; 1–

10 percent of men and 20–40 percent of women remain asymptomatic; asymptomatically infected persons accumulate in population; therefore, among cases diagnosed by screening or testing of named sexual contacts, up to 90 percent may be asymptomatic; most rectal and pharyngeal infections remain asymptomatic

Symptoms Primarily urethral or vaginal discharge; dysuria, usually without urgency or frequency; intermenstrual bleeding or menorrhagia; proctitis causes anal discharge, pruritus, occasionally tenesmus and rectal bleeding; major symptoms of complicated gonorrhea are low abdominal pain, testicular pain and swelling, polyarthralgias, skin lesions, conjunctival pain and discharge, constitutional symptoms

Epidemiologic History New sex partner; high-risk partner; demographic markers of risk (see above)

PHYSICAL EXAMINATION

Men Urethral discharge, usually overt but sometimes demonstrated only by "milking" penis; discharge typically yellow, but less purulent exudate (mucoid, white) sometimes seen; occasionally penile edema or lymphangitis; may be normal

Women Purulent or mucopurulent endocervical exudate or other signs of mucopurulent cervicitis (see Chap. 17); sometimes purulent exudate expressed from urethra, periurethral (Skene's) glands, or Bartholin gland duct; sometimes uterine or adnexal tenderness or mass (see Chap. 19); may be normal

Proctitis Usually normal; occasional perianal erythema; anoscopy may show mucosal erythema, punctate bleeding, purulent exudate

Pharyngeal Infection Usually normal; occasional erythema; rare purulent exudate, cervical lymphadenopathy

LABORATORY DIAGNOSIS

Gram-Stained Smear Smear of exudate typically shows PMNs with intracellular gram-negative diplococci (ICGND); highly reliable in symptomatic urethritis; for cervical, rectal, or asymptomatic urethral infection, smear detects only about 50 percent of cases, but positive result in experienced hands is a reliable indicator of gonorrhea; not useful for pharyngeal infection

Culture Culture all symptomatic and exposed sites; culture detects 95–100 percent of symptomatic male urethral infections and 80–90 percent of cervical, rectal, or pharyngeal infections; immediate inoculation of culture plate is ideal, but most transport media acceptable if processed within 6 hours; do not refrigerate specimen after collection

Other Tests All available nonculture tests are less sensitive or less specific than culture and do not preserve organism for antimicrobial susceptibility testing; do not use unless culture unavailable; no useful serologic test

TREATMENT

Principles *N. gonorrhoeae* strains with relative or absolute resistance to penicillin and the tetracyclines cause at least 15 percent of gonococcal strains in all parts of United States and >50 percent in some areas; the penicillins are no longer recommended for routine treatment; also avoid tetracyclines as sole treatment; use an effective single-dose regimen plus therapy to eradicate concomitant *Chlamydia trachomatis* infection; sequential treatment may also reduce selection of antibiotic-resistance gonococci; also treat suspected (unconfirmed) cases and exposed sexual partners

Uncomplicated Gonorrhea in Adults
INITIAL TREATMENT

- Ceftriaxone 250 mg IM (single dose); 125 mg considered acceptable by some authorities
- Alternatives (some not reliable for pharyngeal infection): Spectinomycin 2.0 g IM; cefixime 400–800 mg PO; cefotaxime 1.0 g IM; ceftizoxime 500 mg IM; cefuroxime axetil 1.0 g PO plus probenecid 1.0 g PO; ciprofloxacin 500 mg PO; norfloxacin 800 mg PO; ofloxacin 400 mg PO

FOLLOW-UP THERAPY

- Doxycycline 100 mg PO BID for 7 days
- Alternatives: Tetracycline HCl 500 mg PO QID for 7 days; erythromycin 2.0 g/day PO in divided doses for 7 days

Pediatric Gonorrhea (<13 Years Old)
Ceftriaxone 125 mg IM (single dose); increase to 250 mg if body weight ≥100 lb (45 kg); treat gonococcal conjunctivitis or other complications IV or IM for ≥7 days; follow-up treatment usually not given unless *C. trachomatis* documented

Follow-up Repeat culture optional if recommended regimens used and patient adheres to follow-up therapy; women should be rescreened for possible reinfection 4–6 weeks after treatment

CONTROL MEASURES

Management of Sex Partners Notify and treat all partners in 2–4 weeks prior to acquisition; health department may assist in locating partners, especially for complicated cases (e.g., PID)

Screening Routinely screen high-risk persons, especially sexually active women in high-prevalence settings

Reporting Required by law in all states; for special cases (e.g., complications, pediatric infection), promptly telephone health department

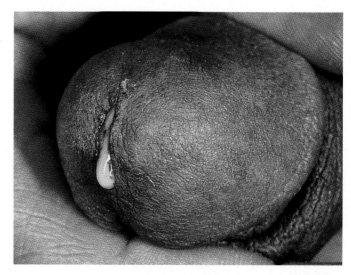

2-1 *Gonococcal urethritis.*

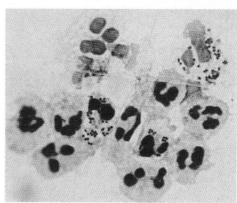

2-2 *Gonococcal urethritis: Gram-stained smear of urethral exudate showing intracellular gram-negative diplococci.*

Patient Profile   Age 22, carwash attendant, IV drug user

History   Urethral discharge for 1 day, mild dysuria; intercourse with a new partner 3 days earlier and regular girlfriend the next night

Examination   Copious purulent urethral discharge; otherwise normal

Differential Diagnosis   Gonorrhea, nongonococcal urethritis

Laboratory   PMNs with ICGND on urethral smear; cultures sent for *N. gonorrhoeae* (reported positive after 2 days) and *C. trachomatis* (positive); syphilis serology; HIV antibody testing and counseling

Diagnosis   Gonococcal urethritis (with chlamydial infection)

Treatment   Ceftriaxone 250 mg IM plus doxycycline 100 mg PO BID for 7 days

Management of Partners   Patient advised to inform and refer both his new partner and girlfriend for treatment

Other   Advised to adhere to doxycycline regimen and abstain from intercourse until treatment completed; told to expect symptomatic improvement within 1–2 days and complete resolution over 4–7 days; case report telephoned to local health department; follow-up scheduled for posttest HIV counseling; counseled regarding prevention of further episodes and risk reduction for all STDs (monogamy, condoms)

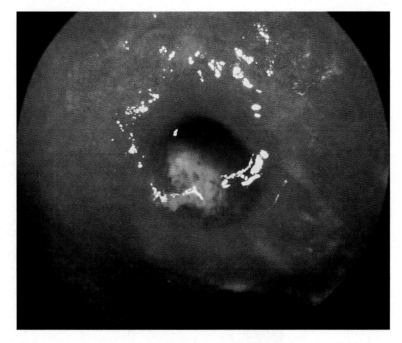

2-3 *Gonococcal cervicitis, with scant purulent exudate in os.* (Courtesy of King K. Holmes, M.D., Ph.D.)

Patient Profile Age 18, unemployed girlfriend of above patient

History Asymptomatic; confirmed exposure 2 days earlier; no other sex partners in past 4 months; had "severe hives" immediately after receiving penicillin 3 years earlier

Examination Mucopurulent cervical exudate; otherwise normal

Laboratory Gram stain of cervical exudate showed PMNs without apparent pathogens; cervical cultures for *N. gonorrhoeae* from cervix (reported as positive 2 days later), anal canal (positive), and pharynx (negative); cervical culture for *C. trachomatis* (positive); VDRL and HIV serology (negative)

Diagnosis Gonococcal cervicitis (with chlamydial infection)

Treatment Spectinomycin 2.0 g IM once plus doxycycline 100 mg PO BID for 7 days; ceftriaxone and other cephalosporins contraindicated by history of immediate penicillin allergy; ciprofloxacin 500 mg or norfloxacin 800 mg PO would be acceptable if oral therapy desired

Management of Sex Partner Already treated

Other Positive rectal culture does not alter management; case report submitted to health department; scheduled for HIV posttest counseling after 7 days and rescreening for gonorrhea and *C. trachomatis* after 4–6 weeks

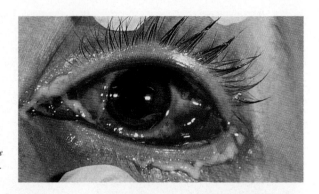

2-4 *a. Gonococcal conjunctivitis; compare with chlamydial conjunctivitis (Fig. 3-3).*

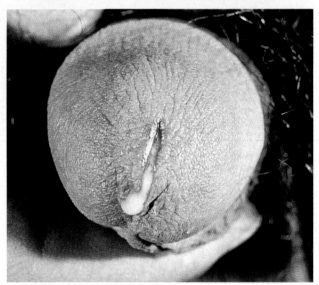

b. Gonococcal urethritis.

Patient Profile   Age 18, homosexual male waiter

History   Urethral discharge for 3 days; left eye pain and photophobia for 1 day

Examination   Conjunctival erythema, purulent exudate, subconjunctival hemorrhage; purulent urethral discharge

Differential Diagnosis   Conjunctivitis due to *N. gonorrhoeae*, HSV, *C. trachomatis*, other pyogenic bacteria

Laboratory   PMNs with ICGND in both conjunctival and urethral exudate; *N. gonorrhoeae* isolated from both sites; urethral and conjunctival cultures for *C. trachomatis* (negative)

Diagnosis   Gonococcal conjunctivitis

Treatment   Ceftriaxone 250 mg IM plus cefixime 400 mg PO once daily for 7 days

Management of Sex Partner(s)   Advised to refer partner(s) for evaluation and treatment

Comment   Compare with chlamydial conjunctivitis (Fig. 3-3); gonococcal conjunctivitis should be treated for $\geq$7 days; although chlamydial co-infection could not be excluded when treatment started, isolation of *C. trachomatis* is relatively uncommon in homosexual men compared with heterosexuals

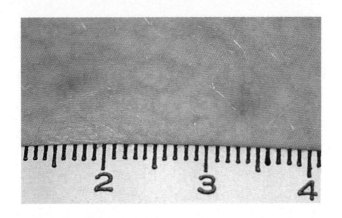

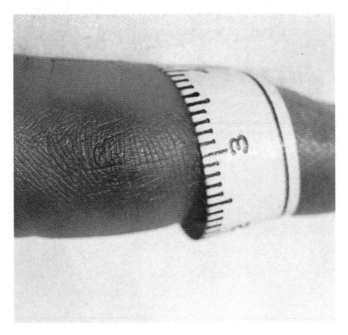

2-5 *Skin lesions in gonoccal arthritis-dermatitis syndrome. a. Early papular lesions of forearm. b. Hemorrhagic lesion of finger. c. Pustule with central eschar. d. Large hemorrhagic pustule of foot. (Parts a and b are from the patient described;*

Patient Profile Age 22, female "exotic dancer" in a bar

History Generalized arthralgias and "red bumps" on arms and legs for 2 days; swelling and pain of several joints for 1 day, preventing dancing; intermittent vaginal discharge, without recent change; currently menstruating; refuses to give information about sex partners

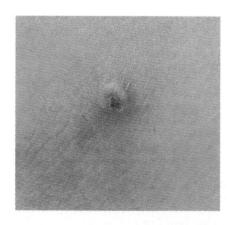

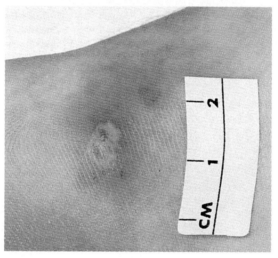

2-5 (continued)   c *and* d *are from two other patients.) Lesions typically begin as nonspecific papules or petechial, then progress to pustules, often with a hemorrhagic component. Pustules may have a central eschar where gonococci initially lodge. The rulers are metric.*

Examination   Afebrile; 15–20 papular, pustular, and hemorrhagic lesions on extremities; slight erythema and edema over left wrist, extending to dorsum of hand; pain on range of motion of left ankle, without visible abnormality; moderate effusion of right knee, with 20 ml slightly cloudy straw-colored fluid obtained by needle aspiration; genital examination showed menstrual blood in vaginal vault, otherwise normal; normal cardiac examination

Differential Diagnosis   Disseminated gonococcal infection, hepatitis B prodrome, other immune complex syndromes, bacterial endocarditis, Reiter's syndrome, acute rheumatic fever, systemic lupus erythematosus, etc.

Laboratory Cervical Gram stain showed few PMNs, no ICGND; synovial fluid contained 8500 leukocytes per mm^3 with 80 percent PMNs, no crystals, no bacteria by Gram stain; cultures for *N. gonorrhoeae* obtained from cervix, anal canal, pharynx, synovial fluid, and blood ($\times$3); routine screening tests done for *C. trachomatis* and syphilis (negative); HIV testing recommended but declined by patient; *N. gonorrhoeae* isolated from cervix and pharynx, other cultures negative

Diagnosis Gonococcal arthritis-dermatitis syndrome

Treatment Hospitalized and treated with ceftriaxone 1.0 g IV once daily

Management of Sex Partners In response to telephoned case report, health department counselor reinterviewed patient in hospital to identify partner(s)

Comment Onset of disseminated gonococcal infection during or near menses is typical; synovial fluid cultures usually are negative in polyarthritis-dermatitis phase of disseminated gonorrhea; close monitoring of cardiac status is indicated for first 2–3 days, because 1–3 percent of patients have gonococcal endocarditis; prompt reporting is essential; patient improved rapidly, discharged after 3 days on ciprofloxacin 500 mg PO BID for 7 days (10 days total treatment)

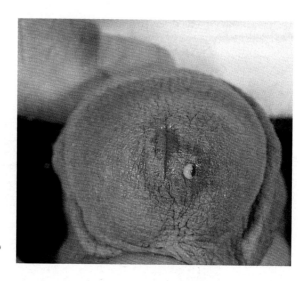

2-6 *Periurethral furuncle due to* Neisseria gonorrhoeae.

Patient Profile   Age 26, heterosexual engineer

History   "Pimple" at tip of penis for 2–3 months, draining pus for 2 days; no dysuria or urethral discharge; in a monogamous relationship for 2 years

Examination   Mildly tender, 6 mm erythematous papule adjacent to meatus; purulent discharge expressed, with scant bleeding; no urethral exudate or lymphadenopathy

Differential Diagnosis   Furuncle, infected sebaceous cyst, pyderma; STD seemed unlikely, based on reliable history of monogamy

Laboratory   Gram stain of lesion exudate showed many PMNs with rare ICGND; urethral smear normal; lesion culture sent for *N. gonorrhoeae,* reported positive 3 days later, confirmed by sugar utilization reactions; urethral cultures for *N. gonorrhoeae* and *C. trachomatis,* both negative; syphilis and HIV serology negative

Diagnosis   Gonococcal furuncle or periurethral gland infection

Treatment   Cefixime 800 mg PO, single dose

Management of partners   Further history revealed that patient's partner frequently traveled to Hawaii on business and returned from most recent trip 3 months earlier, 1 week before onset of lesion; partner subsequently admitted to intercourse with other partners during business trips; *N. gonorrhoeae* isolated from cervix

Other Illustrates importance of considering gonorrhea and other STDs in patients with atypical syndromes and not apparently at risk; follow-up treatment with doxycyline deferred because *C. trachomatis* not isolated; lesion had resolved when patient reexamined 10 days after treatment

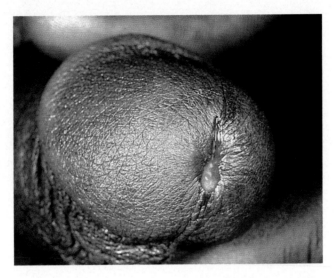

2-7 *Mucopurulent exudate in gonococcal urethritis; not all cases have opaque, overtly purulent discharge (compare with Figs. 2-1 and 2-4b).*

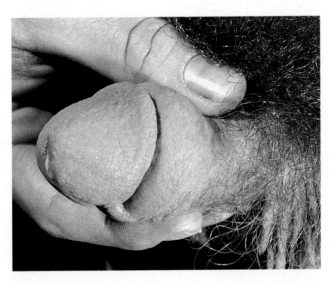

2-8 *Gonococcal urethritis with distal penile cellulitis ("bull-headed clap"). This rare complication of gonorrhea is similar to "penile venereal edema" (Fig. 14-2).*

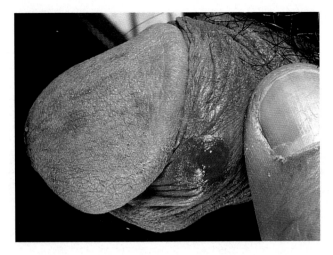

2-9 *Presumptive gonococcal ulcer of the penis in a patient with gonococcal urethritis.* Neisseria gonorrhoeae *rarely can cause genital ulceration, but many cases probably represent secondary gonococcal infection of preexisting skin lesions. Workup of this patient for herpes, syphilis, and chancroid was negative and the ulcer healed promptly following treatment for gonorrhea.*

ADDITIONAL READING

Handsfield HH et al: Localized outbreak of penicillinase-producing *Neisseria gonorrhoeae:* Paradigm for introduction and spread of gonorrhea in a community. *JAMA* 261:2357, 1989.

Hook EW III, Handsfield HH: Gonococcal infections in the adult, in *Sexually Transmitted Diseases,* 2d ed, KK Holmes et al (eds). New York, McGraw-Hill, 1990, chap 14.

Moran JS, Zenilman JM: Therapy for gonococcal infections: Options in 1989. *Rev Infect Dis* 12(suppl 6):S633, 1990.

Scwarcz SK et al: National surveillance of antimicrobial resistance in *Neisseria gonorrhoeae. JAMA* 264:1413, 1990.

Chapter 3   Chlamydial Infections

Infection with *Chlamydia trachomatis,* a small bacterium that requires cell culture for isolation, is the most prevalent bacterial STD in industrialized countries and perhaps worldwide. Some serotypes are the cause of blinding trachoma, a continuing public health problem in some developing countries. Three serotypes cause lymphogranuloma venereum (LGV), one of the five classical venereal diseases (with gonorrhea, syphilis, chancroid, and donovanosis). The trachoma and LGV serotypes are now uncommon in industrialized countries. *C. pneumoniae* (until recently known as the "TWAR" agent) is a newly described species and a common cause of respiratory infection; it is not sexually transmitted.

Except for LGV, the clinical spectrum of genital chlamydial infection is similar to that of gonorrhea, but with less florid symptoms and signs, a longer incubation period, and more frequent asymptomatic infection. Recent data have confirmed the longstanding clinical impression that inapparent genital chlamydial infection can become clinically manifest after intervals as long as several years. Paradoxically, the outwardly mild nature of chlamydial infection may enhance the frequency of complications, because treatment is often delayed and significant scarring (e.g., fallopian tube obstruction) can result from minimally symptomatic or asymptomatic infection. Difficulties in clinical recognition and diagnosis have seriously hampered efforts at prevention and control of chlamydial infection, as has failure to implement widespread routine screening, partner notification, and related control measures.

EPIDEMIOLOGY

Incidence and Prevalence   Overall incidence in industrialized countries estimated at 3–4 times that of gonorrhea; prevalence 5–10 times that of gonorrhea in some settings (e.g., women attending family planning clinics, private physicians' offices); 10–20 percent of patients in most STD clinics are infected; LGV rare in United States (277 cases reported in 1990)

Transmission   Exclusively by sexual contact or perinatally, except for transmission of trachoma strains among children

Age   Reflects sexual behavior patterns; rapidly decreasing prevalence in women after age 25, perhaps due to acquired immunity as well as modified sexual behavior

Sex   Distribution reflects behavioral patterns in community

Race   More common in black, Hispanic, and Native American than white and Asian populations in the United States, but these racial differences are less than for gonorrhea

Sexual Orientation   Now relatively uncommon in homosexually active men; presumably rare in exclusively homosexual women

Other Risk Factors   Most common in populations of low socioeconomic and education level, but these markers are less predictive than for gonorrhea; some reports suggest birth control pills may increase risk (controversial); common in all populations

HISTORY

Incubation Period Usually 1–3 weeks; many infections remain asymptomatic

Symptoms Urethral or vaginal discharge, dysuria; other symptoms of urethritis, mucopurulent cervicitis, PID, epididymitis, or conjunctivitis (see Chaps. 2, 14–19)

Epidemiologic History Presence of STD risk factors and markers enhances risk, but infection is common in their absence

PHYSICAL EXAMINATION

Findings of urethritis, cervicitis, salpingitis, proctitis, epididymitis, and other manifestations (see Chaps. 14–19)

LABORATORY DIAGNOSIS

Culture Isolation in cell culture the diagnostic standard, but availability limited and cost high

Nonculture Tests Direct immunofluorescence microscopy using monoclonal antibody (e.g., MicroTrak), enzyme immunoassay (e.g., Chlamydiazyme), or other technologies; less sensitive than culture but more widely available and less expensive; other methodologies under investigation, including genetic detection; nonculture tests approved only for urethra, cervix, and conjunctivae; not recommended for test-of-cure

because antigens may persist despite killing of organism

Serology Helps in diagnosis of LGV (complement fixation titer $\geq 1:128$); rarely useful in other settings, except for research

TREATMENT

Treatment of Choice Doxycycline 100 mg PO BID for 7 days

Alternative Regimens Tetracycline hydrochloride 500 mg PO QID for 7 days; erythromycin 2.0 g PO in divided doses for 7 days; sulfamethoxazole 1.0 g PO BID for 7–10 days (or equivalent sulfonamide regimen); high-dose amoxicillin has modest efficacy, if other regimens contraindicated; probable role for single-dose therapy with azithromycin, a new long-acting macrolide-like antibiotic (1.0 g PO)

CONTROL MEASURES

Management of Sex Partners Notify and treat partners at risk (usually all partners in preceding 1–2 months)

Screening Routinely screen sexually active younger women; one useful approach is to test all with 2 or more of following characteristics: age ≤ 25 years, new partner in preceding 2 months, abnormal cervical exudate, endocervical bleeding with gentle swabbing, and use of no contraception or a nonbarrier method; routine testing may be warranted for males in some settings (e.g., STD clinics, juvenile detention clinics)

Reporting Promptly report cases where required by local regulations

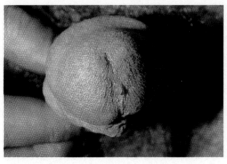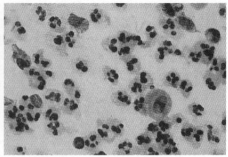

3-1 *Nongonococcal urethritis due to* Chlamydia trachomatis. *a. Mucopurulent urethral discharge (also see Fig. 14-1). b. Gram-stained urethral smear showing PMNs without ICGND.* (Courtesy of Walter E. Stamm, M.D.)

Patient Profile   Age 19, single heterosexual college sophomore

History   Began new sexual relationship 6 weeks earlier; no other partners for 6 months; intermittent urethral discharge without dysuria during past 3 weeks; referred by partner after she had positive screening test for *C. trachomatis* at local family planning clinic

Examination   Scant mucoid urethral discharge, manifested primarily by urethral moisture (patient had not urinated for >4 hours)

Differential Diagnosis   Chlamydial urethritis, nonchlamydial NGU; gonorrhea, trichomonal, and herpetic urethritis are less likely

Laboratory   Urethral Gram stain showed 10–15 PMNs per 1000× field, without ICGND; culture for *C. trachomatis* (positive) and *N. gonorrhoeae* (negative); VDRL and serologic test for HIV (both negative)

Diagnosis   Chlamydial NGU

Treatment   Doxycycline 100 mg PO BID for 7 days

Other   Mild symptoms and subtle clinical findings typical of chlamydial infection; counseled to use condoms for all sexual exposures

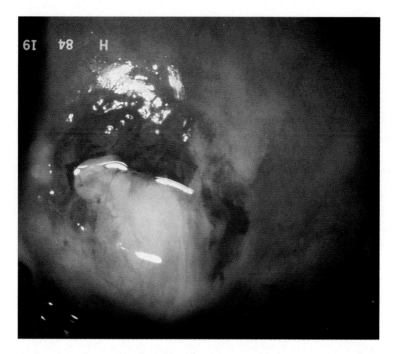

3-2   *Mucopurulent cervicitis due to* Chlamydia trachomatis (*see also Figs.* 8-6, 17-1, 17-3, 17-4, *and* 17-5). (Courtesy of Claire E. Stevens.)

Patient Profile   Age 23, female prostitute

History   Asymptomatic; presented for routine STD screening every 3–4 months

Examination   Small area of cervical ectopy with moderate mucopurulent exudate in os and capillary fragility; otherwise normal

Differential Diagnosis   Possible mucopurulent cervicitis (chlamydial, gonococcal, other)

Laboratory   Cervical Gram stain showed 15–20 PMNs per 1000× field, without ICGND; pH 4.0; negative KOH amine odor test; no yeasts, clue cells, or trichomonads seen microscopically; cultures sent for *C. trachomatis* (positive) and *N. gonorrhoeae* (negative); serologic tests for syphilis and HIV (negative)

Diagnosis   Asymptomatic chlamydial cervicitis

Treatment   Doxycycline 100 mg PO BID for 7 days

Management of Partners   Advised to refer identifiable partners in preceding 2 months for examination and treatment

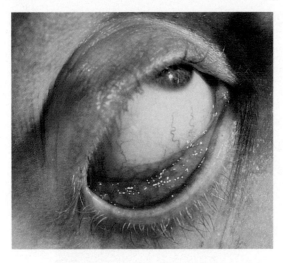

3-3 *Chlamydial conjunctivitis; compare with gonococcal conjunctivitis (Fig. 2-4).*

Patient Profile   Age 22, female flight attendant

History   Boyfriend with NGU; mild itching of right eye for 2–3 weeks

Examination   Slight conjunctival erythema with hypertrophied "cobblestone" appearance; genital examination showed mucopurulent cervicitis

Differential Diagnosis   Conjunctivitis due to *C. trachomatis, N. gonorrhoeae, Haemophilus* sp., other pyogenic bacteria, viruses, or allergy

Laboratory   Gram-stained conjunctival smear negative; *C. trachomatis* isolated from conjunctival scraping and cervix

Diagnosis   Chlamydial conjunctivitis

Treatment   Doxycycline 100 mg PO BID for 7 days

Comment   Typical chlamydial conjunctivitis; this case and Fig. 2-4 illustrate generic differences between gonorrhea and chlamydial infection with respect to incubation period, acuteness, and severity of inflammatory signs; the differences are similar for all anatomic sites

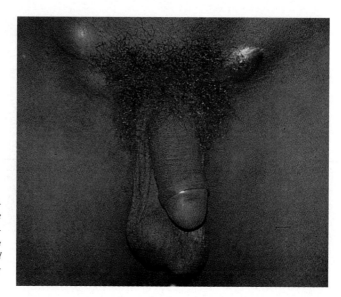

3-4 *Lymphogranuloma venereum. Note the separation of right lymph nodes by the inguinal ligament ("groove sign"). The lesion on the patient's left had ruptured and partially drained.* (Courtesy of Professor Olu Osoba.)

Patient Profile Age 27, unmarried man who immigrated from Ethiopia 3 weeks earlier; prior to immigration, visited prostitutes 3–4 times per month

History Painful swellings in groin for 2 weeks; no other symptoms

Examination Moderately tender, firm inguinal lymphadenopathy bilaterally; nodes divided by inguinal ligament on left; no other lymphadenopathy; otherwise normal

Differential Diagnosis Syphilis, lymphogranuloma venereum, HIV infection, cat-scratch disease, pyogenic or mycobacterial infection, lymphoma

Laboratory Urethral Gram stain negative for PMNs and ICGND; urethral cultures for *N. gonorrhoeae, C. trachomatis* (both negative); serologic tests for syphilis and HIV (negative); chlamydia/LGV complement fixation test reactive, titer 1:1024

Diagnosis Lymphogranuloma venereum

Treatment Doxycycline 100 mg PO BID for 3 weeks

Comment Absence of detectable cutaneous primary lesion or urethritis is typical; division of involved lymph nodes by inguinal ligament ("groove" sign) is common in LGV; patient requires weekly follow-up, with needle aspiration if lymph nodes become fluctuant; scheduled for repeat VDRL after 3 months and HIV serology after 3 and 6 months

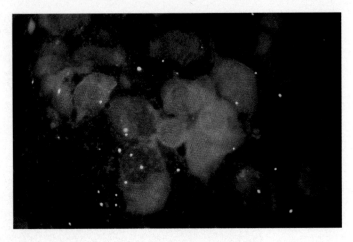

3-5 *Direct immunofluorescence stain of* Chlamydia trachomatis *in an endocervical smear.* C. trachomatis *elementary bodies show bright apple-green fluorescence; host cells are counterstained red.* (Courtesy of Walter E. Stamm, M.D.)

ADDITIONAL READING

Batteiger BE, Jones RB: Chlamydial infections. *Infect Dis Clin North Am* 1:55, 1987.

Handsfield HH et al: Criteria for selective screening for *Chlamydia trachomatis* infection in women attending family planning clinics. *JAMA* 255:1730, 1986.

Stamm WE: Diagnosis of *Chlamydia trachomatis* genitourinary infections. *Ann Intern Med* 108:710, 1988.

Stamm WE, Holmes KK: *Chlamydia trachomatis* infections of the adult, in *Sexually Transmitted Diseases,* 2d ed, KK Holmes et al (eds). New York, McGraw-Hill, 1990, chap 16.

Toomey KE, Barnes RC: Treatment of *Chlamydia trachomatis* genital infection. *Rev Infect Dis* 12(suppl 6):S645, 1990.

Chapter 4   Syphilis

Syphilis has been recognized since the late fifteenth century. It is characterized by a complex course that is largely determined by the unique character of the causative spirochete, *Treponema pallidum,* and the immunologic response to it. Syphilis is classically described as having clinically distinct primary, secondary, and tertiary stages that occur over several years or decades, interspersed by periods of inactive ("latent") infection. However, these distinctions are often blurred, and some manifestations usually considered part of the spectrum of tertiary infection (e.g., neurosyphilis) in fact are most common in early syphilis. Close interactions occur between syphilis and infection with human immunodeficiency virus. HIV may adversely affect the natural course of syphilis or reduce the therapeutic efficacy of penicillin, especially if the central nervous system is involved. Conversely, the presence of lesions caused by *T. pallidum,* like other genital ulcers, appears to enhance the transmission of HIV.

In the late 1980s, the incidence of syphilis in the United States rose rapidly in most urban areas. The populations at maximal risk are those with high incidences of illicit drug use and prostitution. The shift from predominantly homosexual male transmission in the 1970s and early 1980s to heterosexual transmission among socioeconomically disadvantaged populations has been associated with rapidly rising rates of congenital syphilis, the most devastating form of the disease.

EPIDEMIOLOGY

Incidence and Prevalence   In the United States 51,000 cases of primary and secondary syphilis reported in 1990 (87 percent higher than in 1985)

Transmission   Sexually transmissible only during primary, secondary, and early-latent stages; congenital syphilis results from transplacental infection

Age   Early syphilis rates consistent with ages of maximal sexual activity; late manifestations occur at any age

Sex   Distribution reflects patterns of sexual activity; male:female ratio currently 1.4:1 in the United States

Race   In the United States, incidence 5- to 25-fold higher in black, Hispanic, and Native American populations than whites or Asians; race is an indirect marker for societal and behavioral risks

Sexual Orientation   Greatly increased risk in homosexual and bisexual men in 1970s and early 1980s, now lower; apparently rare in exclusively homosexual women

Other Risk Factors   Urban residence; illicit drug use; prostitution or sexual exposure to prostitutes; unmarried; other indirect markers of behavioral risks

CLINICAL MANIFESTATIONS

Epidemiologic History   Sexual partner with syphilis or compatible symptoms; anonymous partner; regular partner known or suspected to have other sexual partners; other epidemiologic risk markers

Incubation Period   Usually 2–6 weeks, occasionally up to 3 months

Symptoms and Signs

PRIMARY SYPHILIS   Chancre usually presents as a single painless or minimally painful round or oval ulcer, typically indurated, often with little or no visible purulent exudate; regional lymphadenopathy is common, usually bilateral, with firm, nonfluctuant, nontender or mildly tender nodes; usually no systemic symptoms; asymptomatic infections are common, probably due to unrecognized chancres; all clinical manifestations and course may be highly variable, and atypical cases are common

SECONDARY SYPHILIS Protean manifestations; most common presentation is generalized, papulosquamous, nonpruritic skin rash, typically involving palms and soles; atypical rashes, including pruritic ones, may occur; other common manifestations include mucous patches (painless mucous membrane lesions), condylomata lata (genital or perianal warty excrescences), patchy alopecia, generalized lymphadenopathy, fever, headache, malaise; focal neurologic manifestations (especially cranial nerve abnormalities) occur occasionally

TERTIARY (LATE) SYPHILIS   Classical tertiary syphilis now rare; most common features are gummas (locally destructive lesions involving the liver, skin, bones, or other organs); late neurosyphilis (tabes dorsalis, general paresis); cardiovascular infection, especially ascending aortic aneurysm and aortic valvular insufficiency

LATENT SYPHILIS Asymptomatic infection, only detectable serologically; arbitrarily divided into early-latent and late-latent stages (<1 year and ≥1 year after infection, respectively)

CONGENITAL SYPHILIS   Severity ranges from asymptomatic to fatal; common early manifestations include spontaneous abortion, stillbirth, encephalitis, generalized skin rash, rhinitis ("snuffles"), hepatic dysfunction, consumption coagulopathy, multiple organ failure; other manifestations, often not apparent at birth, include osteitis of long bones, dental malformations, keratitis, neurosensory hearing loss, chronic neuropsychological deficits, others

LABORATORY DIAGNOSIS

Identification of *T. pallidum*   Cannot be cultivated; detection depends on visual or antigenic identification

DARK-FIELD MICROSCOPY   Motile spirochetes typical of *T. pallidum* in chancre, lymph node aspirate, or moist lesion of secondary syphilis (e.g., condylomata lata); requires careful specimen collection and experienced microscopist; commensal spiral organisms limit utility for oral mucosal lesions

IMMUNOLOGIC DETECTION   Currently available polyclonal fluorescent antibody test is moderately effective substitute for darkfield; much improved monoclonal antibody methods may be available in future

HISTOLOGY   Silver stain or immunofluorescence in tissue specimens; insensitive but sometimes diagnostic in biopsied lesions

Serology   Mainstay of laboratory diagnosis in most settings

NONTREPONEMAL TESTS   Venereal Disease research Laboratory (VDRL) test and variants, including rapid plasma reagin (RPR); detects antibody to "cardiolipin," a component of normal mammalian cell membranes; sensitive but nonspecific; positives require confirmation with specific treponemal antibody test.

The two major uses of the nontreponemal tests are (1) screening and (2) assessment of disease activity. The VDRL and RPR become reactive during primary syphilis, rising to maximal titer (usually 1:16 to 1:256) in secondary syphilis. The titer falls spontaneously thereafter, typically to 1:1 to 1:8 in late-latent infection, but often rises again if there is progression to tertiary disease. The titer usually declines following successful treatment. For primary and secondary syphilis, it should fall by at least 2 dilutions (e.g., from 1:16 to 1:4) within 3 months of treatment; in >90 percent of patients, the titer will be negative by 12 months. In late syphilis, by contrast, low titers (1:1 to 1:2) often persist after apparently successful treatment. Biological false-positive results (i.e., with negative treponemal test results) occasionally occur, often associated with pregnancy or immunologic disorders; the titer usually is ≤1:8.

TREPONEMAL ANTIBODY TESTS   Tests for specific antibody *T. pallidum,* such as fluorescent treponemal antibody-absorbed (FTA-ABS) test, and various hemagglutination assays, such as the microhemagglutination assay for *T. pallidum* (MHA-TP).

The primary use of the treponemal tests is to confirm the results of the VDRL or RPR. Most treponemal antibody assays are not subject to accurate quantitation. Once reactive, the treponemal tests usually remain positive indefinitely, regardless of clinical stage and treatment; however, they occasionally revert to negative after early syphilis. Regardless of clinical stage, reactive treponemal tests revert to negative in some patients with advanced HIV infection. Once a specific treponemal antibody test is positive, repeat tests rarely are indicated; rather the quantitative nontreponemal assays are used to monitor disease activity.

DIAGNOSIS

Most cases of primary and secondary syphilis are readily suspected on clinical grounds, with laboratory confirmation. The diagnosis of late or latent syphilis is dependent on clinical assessment and serology. Except early in the primary stage, the diagnosis of syphilis is rarely warranted in the absence of a reactive treponemal antibody test.

CEREBROSPINAL FLUID EXAMINATION   Some authors recommend cerebrospinal fluid (CSF) examination for all patients with syphilis >1 year in duration. Unequivocal indications are syphilis >1 year in duration plus any of the following: neurologic signs or symptoms; failure of initial therapy; VDRL or RPR titer ≥1:32; other evidence of active syphilis; HIV infection; or planned treatment with a drug other than penicillin. CSF examination also should be performed and treatment for neurosyphilis given to patients with early syphilis (<1 year in duration) if there are symptoms or signs compatible with neurologic involvement.

HIV AND NEUROSYPHILIS   HIV infection may alter the clinical course and response to treatment of syphilis, especially if *T. pallidum* infects the central nervous system. Some evidence suggests that the CSF should be examined in all HIV-infected patients with syphilis, regardless of duration, stage, and presence or absence of clinical neurologic involvement, and that all HIV-infected patients with CSF abnormalities compatible with neurosyphilis should be treated for neurosyphilis. However, these recommendations are controversial.

TREATMENT

Principles Penicillin G remains the drug of choice for all stages of syphilis. The tetracyclines are somewhat less active but usually are used when penicillin cannot be given. Erythromycin should be used only if compliance and close follow-up are absolutely assured. Ceftriaxone and newer β-lactam antibiotics are active against *T. pallidum* and may have a role in some settings when penicillin cannot be given. The sulfonamides, quinolones, nitroimidazoles, and aminoglycosides are inactive. Antibiotic levels sufficient to inhibit *T. pallidum* must be maintained for ≥10 days for early syphilis and ≥4 weeks for late syphilis.

A substantial minority of patients with early syphilis and a few patients with late syphilis experience Jarisch-Herxheimer reactions, with fever, chills, malaise, headache, and often increased inflammation of the chancre or skin rash. The reaction is believed to result from release of treponemal antigens following rapid killing of *T. pallidum*; it typically begins 6–12 hours after treatment and resolves within 24 hours.

Recommended Regimens

EARLY SYPHILIS—PRIMARY, SECONDARY, AND EARLY-LATENT (<1 YEAR IN DURATION)

Treatment of choice

- Benzathine penicillin G 2.4 million units IM, single dose

Alternative regimens for penicillin-allergic patients

- Doxycycline 100 mg PO BID for 2 weeks
- Tetracycline HCl 500 mg PO QID for 2 weeks

- Erythromycin 500 mg QID PO for 2 weeks (if other regimens unsuitable and compliance and follow-up assured)
- Ceftriaxone 250 mg IM once daily for 10 days (only preliminary data available; use only if other regimens unsuitable and compliance and follow-up assured)

LATE SYPHILIS (>1 YEAR DURATION), EXCEPT NEUROSYPHILIS

Treatment of choice

- Benzathine penicillin G 2.4 million units IM weekly for 3 doses

Alternative regimens

- Doxycycline 100 mg PO BID for 4 weeks
- Tetracycline HCl 500 mg PO QID for 4 weeks

NEUROSYPHILIS

Treatment of choice

- Aqueous penicillin G 2–4 million units IV every 4 hours (12–24 million units daily) for 10–14 days

Outpatient alternative (if compliance assured)

- Procaine penicillin G 2.4 million units IM daily, plus probenecid 500 mg PO QID, for 10–14 days

Additional Therapy Some authorities recommended following either of the above regimens with 3 weekly doses of benzathine penicillin, as for late syphilis without neurologic involvement

Note Only penicillin has been shown to be effective for neurosyphilis; penicillin-allergic patients should be desensitized in consultation with an expert and treated with penicillin

SYPHILIS IN PREGNANT WOMEN Penicillin, appropriate to clinical stage; if allergic, desensitize and treat with penicillin; tetracyclines contraindicated; erythromycin does not treat fetal infection

CONGENITAL SYPHILIS Treatment issues are complex; treat with penicillin in consultation with an expert

Follow-up

EARLY SYPHILIS Reexamine and obtain quantitative VDRL or RPR 1, 3, and 6 months after treatment or until negative; if still reactive, repeat at 6–12 month intervals for 1–2 years

LATE SYPHILIS Reexamine and obtain quantitative VDRL or RPR after 3, 6, and 12 months; repeat at 12-month intervals for 2–3 years if test remains reactive

HIV-INFECTED PATIENTS Reexamine and obtain quantitative VDRL or RPR after 1, 2, and 3 months, then at 3-month intervals for at least 1–2 years or until negative, then yearly (even if negative)

NEUROSYPHILIS Follow as appropriate for stage and HIV status; if CSF abnormal before treatment, repeat CSF examination at 6-month intervals until cell count normal and CSF-VDRL negative

CONTROL MEASURES

Management of Sex Partners Examine and obtain serologic tests for syphilis on all partners exposed during infectious period; treat seronegative partners who have had contact with an infectious case within preceding 3 months, using a regimen effective for primary syphilis; local or state health department usually will assist in identifying and notifying partners

Screening Routine serology for high-risk persons, especially those with characteristics of core transmitters; most states require testing of all pregnant women; in some settings, routine screening may be warranted for all patients seeking care at selected clinics, hospitals, or emergency departments, depending on local epidemiology

Reporting Accurate statistics required to allocate resources, target prevention programs, and provide counseling and partner-notification services; required by law in all states; for suspected primary, secondary, or early-latent syphilis, promptly telephone health department

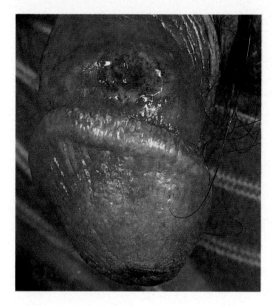

4-1　*Penile chancre in primary syphilis.*

Patient Profile　Age 25, unemployed IV drug user

History　Painless sore on penis for 10 days; frequent intercourse with unnamed women at a local crack house

Examination　Indurated, minimally tender, clean-appearing ulcerative lesion of penis; 2- to 3-cm slightly tender, rubbery inguinal lymph nodes bilaterally

Differential Diagnosis　Syphilis, herpes, chancroid, LGV; nonsexually-transmitted conditions less likely

Laboratory　Dark-field microscopy positive for spirochetes; stat RPR positive; next day, laboratory reported positive VDRL (titer 1:8) and reactive MHA-TP; screening tests done for gonorrhea and *C. trachomatis;* HIV test ordered, with pretest counseling

Diagnosis　Primary syphilis

Treatment　Benzathine penicillin G 2.4 million units IM

Management of Partners　Patient interviewed by health department counselor who obtained first names, descriptions, and other information that led to treatment of two women, one with secondary syphilis

Comment　Typical case; treatment for primary syphilis would be warranted even if dark-field and serologic tests had been negative

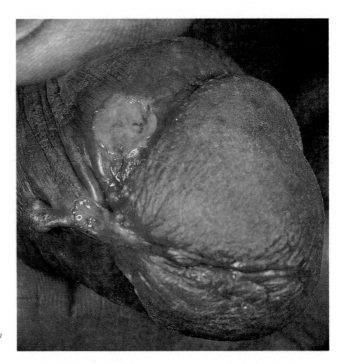

4-2 *Two penile chancres in primary syphilis.*

Patient Profile   Age 32, married assembly line worker with 4-year history of recurrent (every 3–4 months) genital herpes

History   Penile sores 3 weeks; delayed seeking care because "I just thought my herpes was back"; treated 5 years previously for secondary syphilis; occasional anonymous sex with other men in bars or parks, often without condoms

Examination   Two adjacent, indurated, minimally tender penile lesions with clean bases; "shotty" nontender inguinal lymphadenopathy

Differential Diagnosis   Primary syphilis, recurrent herpes; other causes less likely

Laboratory   Dark-field examination of lesion positive for spirochetes; stat RPR positive; culture of lesions for herps simplex virus (later reported negative); VDRL reactive, titer 1:64; HIV serology negative

Diagnosis   Primary syphilis

Treatment   Benzathine penicillin G 2.4 million units IM

Management of Partners   Wife contacted by health department; found to be VDRL-negative, treated with benzathine penicillin G

Other   Patient's history and the presence of 2 lesions suggested possibility of genital herpes; however, multiple chancres occasionally occur in syphilis; MHA-TP or FTA-ABS not indicated, because they are predictably positive owing to patient's prior episode of syphilis; intensively counseled about safer sex and risks associated with anonymous homosexual encounters; advised to have repeat HIV serology after 3 months; patient was referred, at his own request, for counseling to control his compulsive risky sexual behavior

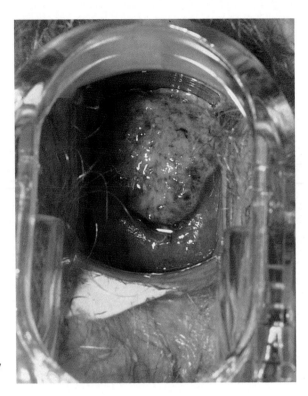

4-3 *Primary syphilis: atypical hypertrophic chancre of cervix.*

Patient Profile Age 24, unmarried clerk-typist

History Partner of a man with secondary syphilis; 2 weeks vaginal discharge, two episodes of postcoital bleeding

Examination Normal external genitalia; prominent exophytic, granular cervical mass that bled readily

Differential Diagnosis Cervical cancer, granulomatous infection (e.g., genital tuberculosis), syphilis

Laboratory Dark-field examination showed motile spirochetes; stat RPR positive; VDRL titer 1:64, FTA-ABS positive; Pap smear showed prominent inflammatory changes; screening tests done for *N. gonorrhoeae, C. trachomatis,* and HIV (all negative)

Diagnosis Atypical, hypertrophic cervical syphilitic lesion, probably primary stage

Treatment   Benzathine penicillin G 2.4 million units IM

Other   Prominent fever and myalgias (Jarisch-Herxheimer reaction) 8 hours after treatment; entirely normal-appearing cervix at 4-week follow-up; illustrates importance of serologic screening for syphilis, because dark-field examination might not have been performed if there were no history of exposure to syphilis

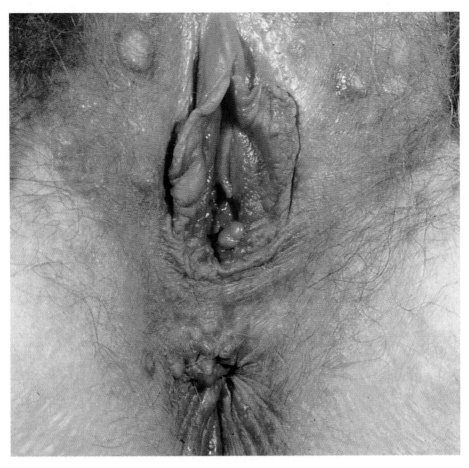

4-4 *Condylomata lata in secondary syphilis; such lesions contain large numbers of* Treponema pallidum (*often dark-field-positive*) *and are highly infectious.*

Patient Profile Age 19, single beautician

History Referred for consultation because of genital and perianal warts for 6 weeks, not responding to repeated weekly applications of podophyllin; past history of urticaria following penicillin therapy; 3 sexual partners in previous 6 months

Examination Several flat, firm, slightly erythematous excrescences of perineum and perianally; bilateral nontender inguinal lymphadenopathy; some perianal lesions ulcerated

Differential Diagnosis Condylomata lata, genital warts

Laboratory Dark-field negative; stat RPR positive; VDRL positive (titer 1:128), MHA-TP reactive

Diagnosis Secondary syphilis with condylomata lata

Treatment Doxycycline 100 mg PO BID for 14 days

Other Lesions resolved within 1 week; illustrates importance of obtaining serologic test for syphilis on all patients with any STD, such as genital warts; interviewed by health department counselor to identify partners

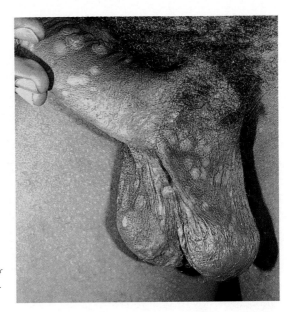

4-11 *Secondary syphilis: papular eruption of penis and scrotum. Depigmented lesions are common in dark-skinned persons.*

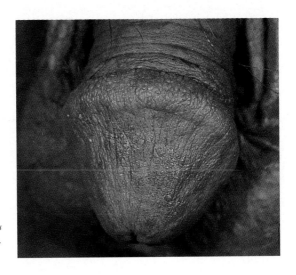

4-12 *Secondary syphilis: papulosquamous rash of penis. Note similarity to scabies (Fig. 13-2) and psoriasis (Figs. 21-3 and 21-4).*

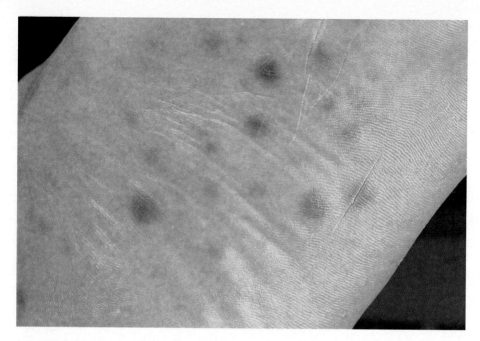

4-13   *Secondary syphilis: papular plantar rash.*

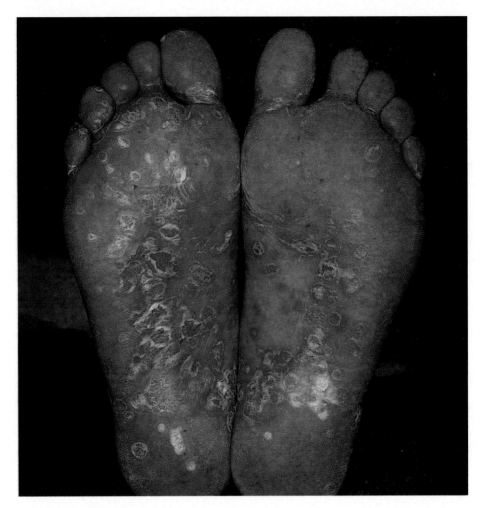

4-14 *Secondary syphilis: extensive hyperkeratotic plantar rash in an HIV-seropositive man with secondary syphilis. Note similarity to keratoderma blenorrhagica of Reiter's syndrome (Fig. 16-3).*

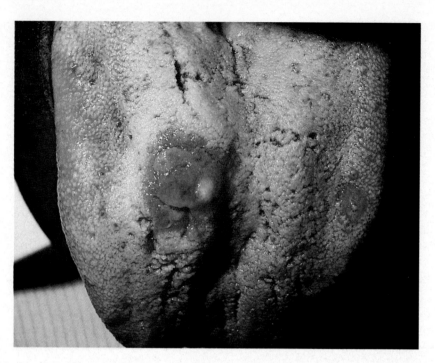

4-15 *Secondary syphilis: mucous patch of tongue. Mucous patches are nontender, usually asymptomatic, but highly infectious.*

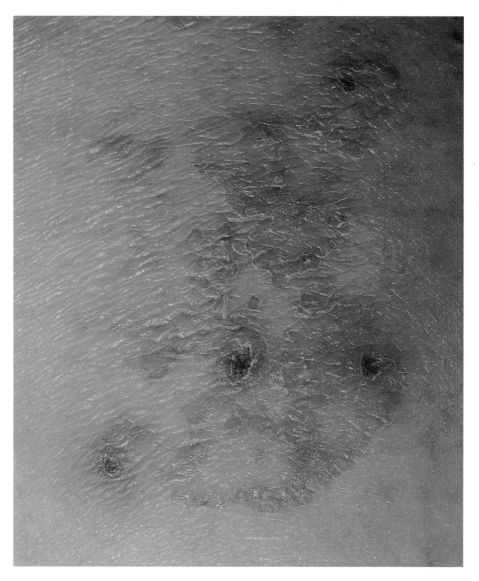

4-16 *Secondary syphilis: atypical eczema-like rash of buttock. Despite its dry appearance, this lesion was dark-field-positive.*

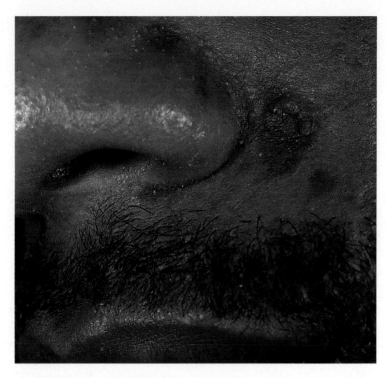

4-17 *Secondary syphilis: hyperpigmented papules of the nose and nasolabial fold. Such lesions are also commonly seen at the corners of the mouth; they often ulcerate and are then called "split papules."*

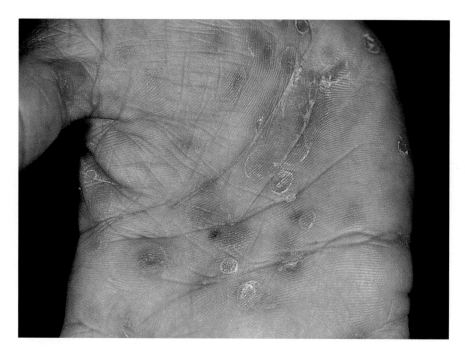

4-18   *Secondary syphilis: palmar rash.*

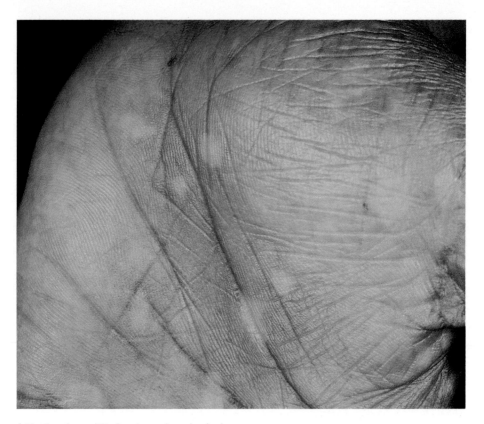

4-19   *Secondary syphilis: hypopigmented macules of palm.*

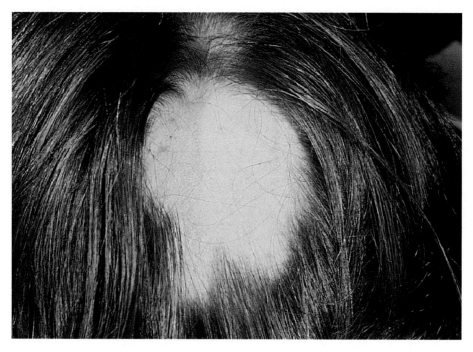

4-20   *Secondary syphilis: alopecia areata of scalp.*

ADDITIONAL READING

Lukehart SA et al: Invasion of the central nervous system by *Treponema pallidum:* Implications for diagnosis and therapy. *Ann Intern Med* 109:855, 1988.

Musher DM et al: Effect of human immunodeficiency virus (HIV) infection on the course of syphilis and on the response to treatment. *Ann Intern Med* 113:872, 1990.

Rolfs RT, Nakashima AK: Epidemiology of primary and secondary syphilis in the United States, 1981–1989. *Jama* 264:1432, 1990.

Sparling PF: Natural history of syphilis, in *Sexually Transmitted Diseases,* 2d ed, KK Holmes et al (eds). New York, McGraw-Hill, 1990, chap 19.

Thin RN: Early syphilis in the adult, in *Sexually Transmitted Diseases,* 2d ed, KK Holmes et al (eds). New York, McGraw-Hill, 1990, chap 20.

Zenker PN, Rolfs RT: Treatment of syphilis, 1989. *Rev Infect Dis* 12(suppl 6):S590, 1990.

Chapter 5   Chancroid

Chancroid is a genital ulcer disease caused by the sexually transmitted bacterium *Haemophilus ducreyi*. It is one of the original five "classical" STDs, along with gonorrhea, syphilis, lymphogranuloma venereum, and donovanosis. On the basis of recent DNA homology studies, it is likely that *H. ducreyi* will be reclassified into a different genus. In most societies, chancroid is more closely linked with prostitution or illicit drug use than are other STDs. This may be explained by the relative infrequency of an asymptomatic carrier state; maintenance of a chancroid outbreak may require a population of persons who have intercourse despite painful genital ulcers. Chancroid has been implicated as an important factor that enhances the sexual transmission of HIV. Reported cases rose rapidly in urban core populations in the United States during the late 1980s.

EPIDEMIOLOGY

Incidence and Prevalence   About 4000–5000 reported cases annually in the United States in 1987–1990, versus a mean of 900 per year in 1980–1984; primarily in urban, ethnic minority populations with high rates of prostitution and illicit drug use

Transmission   Exclusively by sexual contact

Age, Sex, and Race   Reflective of core transmitter populations and patterns of sexual activity

Sexual Orientation   No special predilection

Other Risk Factors   Absence of circumcision enhances risk in men

HISTORY

Incubation Period   Usually 2–10 days

Symptoms   Painful ulceration, sometimes with multiple lesions, usually involving the genitals; inguinal pain and swelling in 50 percent; no systemic symptoms

Epidemiologic History   Sex in setting of prostitution or drug use; recent travel to an endemic area

PHYSICAL EXAMINATION

Tender, nonindurated, genital ulcer(s) with purulent base; surrounding erythema and undermined edges are common; nontender lesions sometimes present; occasionally two to four lesions, sometimes with "kissing" lesions due to apposition of the initial lesion to uninvolved skin; unilateral or bilateral inguinal lymphadenopathy in 50–60 percent; lymphadenopathy is characteristic of pyogenic infection, with erythema, tenderness, often central fluctuance, sometimes spontaneous rupture

LABORATORY DIAGNOSIS

Isolation of *H. ducreyi* from lesion or node aspirate; special media required; sensitivity of culture 60–80 percent, depending on specimen management, variations in media, and laboratory's experience; Gram stain of ulcer may show small gram-negative bacilli, but is insensitive and nonspecific; antigen-detection, genetic, and serologic tests under development; all suspected cases require dark-field microscopic examination, culture for herpes, and serologic test for syphilis

DIAGNOSTIC CRITERIA

Isolation of *H. ducreyi* is definitive; otherwise, diagnosis based on clinical picture, exclusion of genital herpes and syphilis, epidemiologic information (e.g., contact with a case), and response to therapy

TREATMENT

Principles   Many strains of *H. ducreyi* contain β-lactamase plasmids; erythromycin, third-generation cephalosporins, and newer quinolones are uniformly active; sulfamethoxazole/trimethoprim usually active, but some geographic variation; single-dose therapy with ceftriaxone or a quinolone is usually effective, except in patients infected with HIV

Treatments of Choice   Erythromycin 500 mg PO QID for 7 days; or ceftriaxone 250 mg IM (single dose); some authorities administer both regimens

Alternative Regimens   Sulfamethoxazole/trimethoprim 800/160 mg PO BID for 7 days; amoxicillin/clavulanic acid (Augmentin) 500/125 mg PO TID for 7 days (not evaluated in United States, but effective elsewhere); ciprofloxacin 500 mg PO BID for 3 days

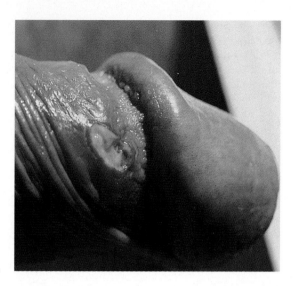

5-1   *Chancroid.*

Patient Profile   Age 26, unmarried salesman

History   Painful sore on penis for 5 days; sexual contact 10 days earlier with a prostitute in a country with high rates of chancroid

Examination   Tender, soft ulcerative penile lesion with purulent base; no lymphadenopathy

Differential Diagnosis   Chancroid, genital herpes, syphilis

Laboratory   Stat RPR and dark-field microscopy negative; culture for HSV (negative); culture for *H. ducreyi* (reported positive 3 days later); tests for urethral chlamydial and gonococcal infection and HIV serology (all negative)

Diagnosis   Chancroid

Treatment   Erythromycin 500 mg PO QID for 7 days; rapid resolution

Comment   Sex partner should be treated as if infected, if she can be identified and located; case report phoned to health department; scheduled for follow-up VDRL after 1 month and repeat HIV serology after 3 and 6 months

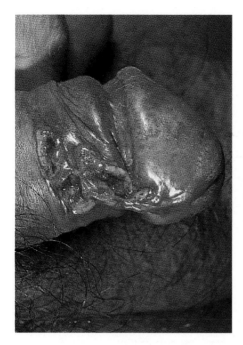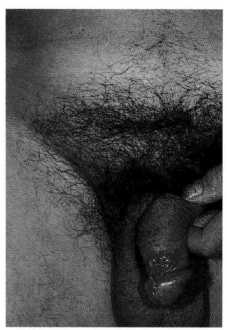

5-2 *Chancroid. a. Penile ulcers. b. Inguinal swelling and erythema.*

Patient Profile Age 60, businessman with a large international corporation

History Painful penile ulcers for 2 weeks, not responding to empiric treatment with amoxicillin; painful right inguinal swelling for 3 days; onset 5 days after sexual contact in an equatorial African country

Examination Multiple irregularly shaped, purulent, tender ulcers under foreskin; 3 × 5 cm indurated, nonfluctuant right inguinal lymph node with overlying erythema extending onto the lower abdominal wall

Differential Diagnosis Classical chancroid; genital herpes, LGV, and syphilis less likely; possible secondary pyogenic infection

Laboratory Dark-field examination and stat RPR negative; lesion cultured for *H. ducreyi* (positive) and HSV (negative); urethral cultures for *N. gonorrhoeae* and *C. trachomatis* (negative); HIV serology (negative)

Diagnosis Chancroid

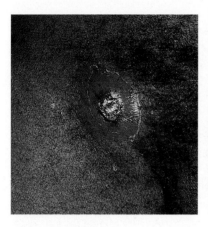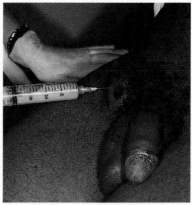

5-3   *a. Fluctuant lymph node in chancroid, with eschar following spontaneous rupture and partial drainage. b. Needle aspiration of lymph node.*

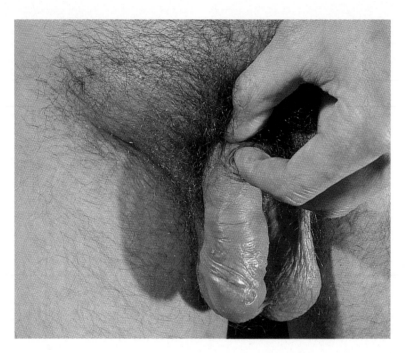

5-4   *Chancroid, with penile ulcers and prominent right inguinal lymphadenopathy with overlying erythema. The eschars adjacent to the lymph node mark the sites of previous needle aspirations.*

II   BACTERIAL SEXUALLY TRANSMITTED DISEASES

Treatment   Ceftriaxone 250 mg IM; because of atypically extensive inguinal erythema and concern about secondary staphylococcal or streptococcal infection, patient was also given amoxicillin with clavulanic acid (Augmentin) 500/125 mg PO TID for 10 days

Management of Sex Partner(s)   Patient advised to notify partner

Comment   Ulcers healed rapidly and cellulitis regressed, but lymph node became fluctuant and required closed-needle drainage 10 days after start of treatment; follow-up syphilis serology scheduled 1 month and repeat HIV serology 3 and 6 months later. Despite numerous visits to his company's travel clinic over several years, the patient—who regularly had sexual exposure while traveling in developing countries—had never been advised to use condoms. Many persons view travel as an opportunity for sexual adventurism, and clinicians who advise travelers should routinely inquire about the potential for sexual exposure, should advise condoms, and should be familiar with the prevalences of STD (including HIV) at common destinations.

ADDITIONAL READING

Krockta WP, Barnes RC: Genital ulceration with regional adenopathy. *Infect Dis Clin North Am* 1:217, 1987.

Ronald AR, Albritton W: Chancroid and *Haemophilus ducreyi,* in *Sexually Transmitted Diseases,* 2d ed, KK Holmes et al (eds). New York, McGraw-Hill, 1990, chap 24.

Schmid GP: Treatment of chancroid, 1989. *Rev Infect Dis* 12(suppl 6):S580, 1990.

Schmid GP et al: Chancroid in the United States: Reestablishment of an old disease. *JAMA* 258:3265, 1987.

Chapter 6 Donovanosis (Granuloma Inguinale)

Donovanosis, or granuloma inguinale, is a rare cause of genital ulcer, even in most developing countries. Endemic foci exist in the Indian subcontinent, Papua New Guinea, and parts of Australia and tropical Africa. Donovanosis is caused by *Calymmatobacterium granulomatis*, a poorly characterized gram-negative bacillus that may be antigenically related to *Klebsiella* sp. The disease is indolent and may be slowly progressive for several years, rarely resulting in autoamputation of the penis. There is rare systemic dissemination, usually manifested by osteolytic lesions.

EPIDEMIOLOGY

Incidence and Prevalence   Rare; usually <50 cases reported annually in the United States.

Transmission   Presumably only by sexual contact; some sexual partners of chronically infected patients remain free of disease for several years

Age, Sex, Race, Sexual Orientation   No known predisposition

HISTORY

Incubation Period   Usually 2 weeks to 3 months

Symptoms   Indolent genital ulcer, often painless; sometimes multiple lesions; chronic cases may be very extensive; occasional inguinal swelling; usually no systemic symptoms

Epidemiologic History   Sexual exposure in an endemic area

PHYSICAL EXAMINATION

One or more genital ulcers with "beefy" base, sometimes hypertrophic, usually without purulent exudate; may mimic carcinoma; tenderness usually absent or mild; "pseudobubo," believed to be the result of subcutaneous extension, may cause inguinal mass mimicking lymphadenopathy, but true lymph node involvement unusual; rarely extensive ulceration lasting several years

LABORATORY DIAGNOSIS

Histologic identification of organism in vacuoles within macrophages ("Donovan bodies") in biopsied tissue or crush preparation from lesion; no known method for consistent isolation of *C. granulomatis*

DIAGNOSTIC CRITERIA

Clinical appearance, plus biopsy or crush preparation showing characteristic histopathology; exposure history; exclusion of other causes of lesion(s)

TREATMENT

Principles Antimicrobial susceptibility only surmised on basis of clinical response to various drugs

Treatments of Choice Tetracycline HCl 500 mg PO QID for 10–21 days, or until healing complete; doxycycline 100 mg PO BID presumably would be effective, but experience limited

Alternative Regimens Sulfamethoxazole/trimethoprim 800/160 mg PO BID has been reported to be effective

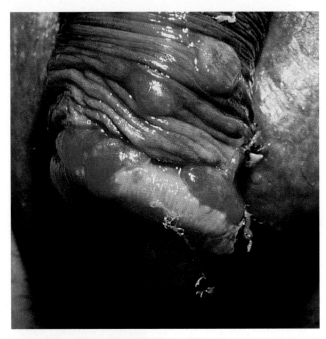

6-1 *Multiple hypertrophic penile ulcers in donovanosis (granuloma inguinale).* (Courtesy of Gavin Hart, M.D.)

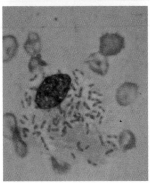

6-2 *Giemsa stain of crush preparation of tissue from a lesion of donovanosis, showing a macrophage containing bipolar-staining bacilli with an appearance suggestive of safety pins ("Donovan bodies").* (Courtesy of Gavin Hart, M.D.)

Patient Profile   Age 47, merchant seaman

History   Painless penile sores for 3 weeks; during 2 months prior to onset had intercourse with several prostitutes in various ports, including coastal cities in India

Examination   Multiple, slightly tender, hypertrophic ulcerative penile lesions; no lymphadenopathy

Differential Diagnosis   Donovanosis, primary syphilis, carcinoma, atypical genital herpes, chancroid, infected traumatic lesions

Laboratory   Negative dark-field microscopy, VDRL, and lesion cultures for HSV and *Haemophilus ducreyi;* negative tests for chlamydial, gonococcal, and HIV infection; histologic examination of ultrathin sections of biopsied tissue from edge of lesion showed large mononuclear cells with Donovan bodies

Diagnosis   Donovanosis

Treatment   Tetracycline HCl 500 mg PO QID for 2 weeks

Management of Sex Partner(s)   Partner(s) should be treated as if infected; impractical in this case

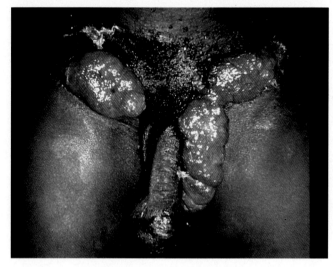

6-3 *Donovanosis. Exuberant granulation tissue with lesions spreading from the penis and scrotum by continuity to one inguinal area, and also to the opposite inguinal area with an intervening skip area, producing pseudobuboes of both inguinal regions.* (Reprinted with permission from KK Holmes et al (eds), *Sexually Transmitted Diseases,* 2d ed. New York, McGraw-Hill, 1990.)

ADDITIONAL READING

Hart G: Donovanosis, in *Sexually Transmitted Diseases,* 2d ed, KK Holmes et al (eds). New York, McGraw-Hill, 1990, chap 25.

Krockta WP, Barnes RC: Genital ulceration with regional adenopathy. *Infect Dis Clin North Am* 1:217, 1987.

Viral Sexually Transmitted Diseases

Chapter 7 Genital Herpes

Genital herpes is the most common cause of genital ulceration in industrialized countries and is among the most common STDs. About 90 percent of genital herpes is caused by herpes simplex virus type 2 (HSV-2), the remainder by type 1 (HSV-1); this ratio is reversed for orolabial herpes, which usually is not acquired sexually. Infection with HSV is lifelong, with the virus persisting in a quiescent (or truly latent) state in dorsal nerve root ganglia. Therefore, the presence of specific antibody denotes current infection and the potential for clinical recurrences and transmission of the virus. Serosurveys suggest that at least 20–25 percent of the U.S. adult population is infected with HSV-2.

Although primary episodes of HSV infection can be severe, recent data suggest that most cases are asymptomatic. However, many apparently asymptomatic infected persons have unrecognized painless or minimally painful lesions, or other manifestations whose significance is not understood. Symptoms often can be ameliorated by systemic treatment with acyclovir, but no cure exists. The most serious complication is neonatal infection, acquired in utero or perinatally, that usually is fatal or causes permanent neurologic sequelae. Genital herpes, like other genital ulcer diseases, appears to be associated with enhanced transmission of HIV.

EPIDEMIOLOGY

Incidence and Prevalence   Recently developed assays that accurately distinguish HSV-1 from HSV-2 antibody demonstrate that 20–30 percent of sexually active young adults in the United States are infected with HSV-2; among patients attending some STD clinics, about 10 percent present with clinically apparent genital herpes, but 50 percent or more are HSV-2 seropositive; annual physician visits for genital herpes in the United States estimated at 100,000 in mid-1970s, rising to 450,000 in late 1980s

Transmission   Only through direct contact with infected lesions or secretions; most transmission occurs from unrecognized lesions or asymptomatic viral shedding, because most patients with overt lesions cease sexual activity; occasional autoinoculation

(e.g., herpetic whitlow, keratoconjunctivitis); transmitted perinatally to newborns

Age   Reflects sexual behavior patterns; most initial cases age 15–30

Sex   No special predilection; symptomatic episodes usually more severe in women than men

Race   Substantially higher seroprevalences in blacks than whites, due to socioeconomic and behavioral factors

Sexual Orientation   High prevalences in homosexual men with multiple partners, in whom anorectal infections are common

Other Risk Factors   Cellular immunodeficiency (e.g., advanced HIV infection) associated with severe manifestations, including chronic, persistent, often debilitating ulcerative lesions

CLINICAL CLASSIFICATION

Primary Herpes   First infection with HSV of either type; seronegative for both HSV-1 and -2 at onset; symptomatic cases commonly severe, prolonged, often with systemic manifestations

First Episode Nonprimary Herpes   First clinical episode in presence of preexisting antibody, usually to opposite HSV type; systemic manifestations uncommon; some cases are first "recurrence" in persons with long-standing subclinical infection

Recurrent Herpes   Repeat clinical episode due to same virus type; large majority of clinical herpes episodes; most cases clinically mild, often evanescent; systemic manifestations rare; usually 2–6 episodes per year

Asymptomatic and Subclinical Herpes Clinically unrecognized chronic infection; may account for half or more of all infections

HISTORY

Incubation Period   Usually 2–10 days (occasionally up to 3 weeks) for symptomatic initial episodes

Symptoms
PRIMARY HERPES   Multiple genital or perianal lesions, usually bilateral or midline; severe pain common in moist areas (e.g., vulva, preputial sac), less painful at drier sites; untreated duration usually 2–3 weeks, but serial crops of lesions may appear over 3–6 weeks; inguinal pain and swelling; dysuria and vaginal or urethral discharge common; neuropathic symptoms referable to sacral nerve roots are common (e.g., urinary retention, constipation, paresthesias); fever, myalgias, malaise, or headache often present; sometimes photophobia, stiff neck

FIRST EPISODE NONPRIMARY HERPES   Fewer lesions than primary infection; may be lateralized, bilateral, or midline; untreated duration 1–2 weeks; inguinal pain and swelling variable; usually no systemic or prominent neuropathic symptoms

RECURRENT HERPES   Few lesions, usually in cluster on only one side of midline; repeated outbreaks usually involve same area of penis, vulva, or buttocks; some patients have prodrome (usually paresthesias) 1–2 days before lesions; lymphadenopathy, systemic symptoms, and overt neuropathy rare; duration usually 7–10 days

SUBCLINICAL HERPES   Usually asymptomatic; some patients have subtle (often painless) lesions, which they ignore

Epidemiologic History   High prevalence in all populations; many patients lack typical high-risk STD profiles; history of exposure or new partner helpful but often absent

PHYSICAL EXAMINATION

Erythematous papules, vesicles, pustules, ulcers, crusts; clusters of lesions are common, especially in recurrent episodes; lesions typically 2–5 mm diameter, but all sizes and shapes occur; usually tender, nonindurated; when present, lymphadenopathy usually is bilateral, firm, moderately tender, without fluctuance or erythema; mucosal lesions common in primary herpes, with erosive cervicitis, urethritis, or proctitis; sacral nerve deficits or meningeal signs may be present

LABORATORY DIAGNOSIS

Viral Isolation   Culture is best test to identify HSV in lesions; now available in most medical centers and laboratories; highest yields from lesions <2 days old; recommended in workup of all etiologically obscure genital ulcers; occasionally useful to detect asymptomatic shedding of HSV from cervix or other sites

Immunologic Detection of HSV Sensitivities of direct fluorescence microscopy and commercial EIA for HSV antigen approach that of culture for ulcerative lesions, but not for detection of asymptomatic shedding

Cytology Tzanck test and other cytologic methods (e.g., Papanicolaou stain) insensitive for ulcerated lesions; often positive for typical vesicular lesions, but rarely useful for atypical or ulcerated lesions

Serology Most commercially available techniques do not reliably distinguish HSV-1 from HSV-2 antibody, despite claims to contrary; newly developed methods are accurate and, when commercially available, will be useful in diagnosis of genital lesions and detection of asymptomatic infection

DIAGNOSTIC CRITERIA

Isolation of HSV or immunologic detection in lesion is definitive, but failure to document HSV usually does not exclude herpes; clinical diagnosis often reliable in typical cases (e.g., clustered vesicles); exclusion of other etiologies (e.g., syphilis, chancroid) important for all clinically atypical cases; obtain syphilis serology for all cases of genital ulcer or lymphadenopathy

TREATMENT

Antiviral Chemotherapy Systemic treatment with acyclovir is mainstay of management of first episode herpes; bioavailability of acyclovir sometimes is poor, and lack of

improvement after 2–3 days oral therapy is an indication to double the dose or switch to IV treatment; topical therapy provides little or no benefit and is rarely indicated

INITIAL (PRIMARY AND NONPRIMARY) GENITAL HERPES

- Usual regimen: Acyclovir 200 mg PO 5 times daily for 7–10 days or until clinical resolution; for dosage convenience, 400 mg TID also is effective

- Primary herpetic proctitis: Acyclovir 400 mg PO 5 times daily (or 800 mg PO TID) for 10 days or until resolution

- Severe cases requiring hospitalization: Acyclovir 5 mg/kg body weight IV every 8 hours for 3–5 days or until improved; then acyclovir PO as above, to complete 10–14 days total therapy

RECURRENT GENITAL HERPES Acyclovir offers little benefit for most cases, but may speed healing in severe cases if started within 1–2 days of onset; some patients with prodromal symptoms may abort outbreaks by prompt self-administered treatment; chronic suppressive therapy reduces recurrences by 75–80 percent, with reduced severity of breakthrough episodes (warn patient that recurrent episodes or transmission may still occur); suppressive treatment usually limited to patients with especially frequent or severe episodes

- Treatment: Acyclovir 200 mg PO 5 times daily (or 400 mg TID) for 5–7 days

- Suppressive therapy: Acyclovir 400 mg PO BID or 200 mg 2–5 times daily; discontinue after 1 year to reassess frequency of recurrences

Supportive Therapy Lesions should be kept clean and dry by washing two to three times daily, wearing loosely fitting cotton underwear, and sprinkling cornstarch in underwear; topical anesthetic ointment may help if labial or meatal lesions make urination difficult

CONTROL MEASURES

Management of Sex Partners Evaluate all partners who do not have prior diagnosis of genital herpes; when available, accurate type-specific serology useful in evaluating asymptomatic partners; educate to recognize any compatible genital lesion and to seek care immediately for diagnosis

Screening Serologic screening with accurate type-specific tests has potential to detect asymptomatically infected persons and thereby to help in counseling to prevent transmission; routine culture or immunologic tests to detect asymptomatic viral shedding in pregnant women near term has little or no value in preventing neonatal infection; presence of maternal lesions at delivery identifies infants at risk of neonatal herpes

Reporting First episode genital herpes and/or neonatal herpes now reportable in several states

Counseling Counsel patient about nature of the infection, potential for recurrences, possibility of asymptomatic viral shedding, and consequent need to warn future sex partners and to use condoms when appropriate

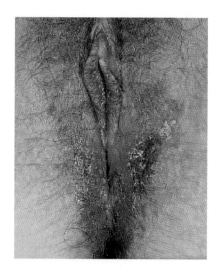

7-1   *Primary genital herpes. a. Multiple ulcerative lesions distributed bilaterally on vulva, labia, and perineum.*

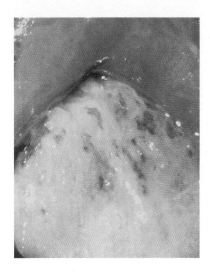

7-1 *(continued)*   *b. Ulcerative herpetic cervicitis (different patient than* a). (Illustration *b* courtesy of Claire E. Stevens.)

Patient Profile   Age 22, single secretary

History   Painful genital lesions, severe dysuria, headache, and fever for 3 days; boyfriend known to have recurrent genital herpes, but they have avoided sexual contact during symptomatic episodes

Examination   Multiple bilateral tender ulcers of labia and introitus; erosive cervicitis; bilateral tender inguinal lymphadenopathy; temperature 38.1°C orally

Differential Diagnosis   Herpes, syphilis, chancroid

Laboratory   HSV-2 isolated from lesions and cervix; syphilis serology, cultures for *N. gonorrhoeae* and *C. trachomatis* (all negative)

Diagnosis   Primary genital herpes

Treatment   Acyclovir 400 mg PO TID for 10 days

Comment   Typical primary herpes; clinical improvement began within 3 days, most lesions healed when examined after 10 days; advised that she can expect recurrences, but much less severe than present episode; over next 14 months, patient had 3 recurrences, each manifested only by a small cluster of lesions that healed rapidly

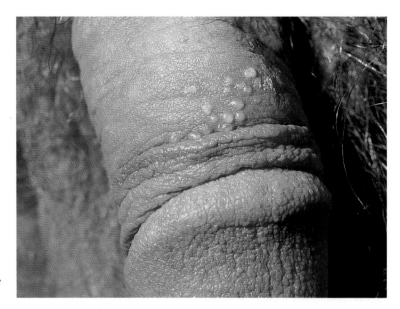

7-2 *Recurrent genital herpes.*

Patient Profile   Age 38, radiology technician

History   Slightly painful penile lesions, preceded by 1 day itching; initial genital herpes diagnosed 2 months previously

Examination   Cluster of pustular lesions at base of penis

Differential Diagnosis   Recurrent genital herpes; pustules also compatible with pyogenic (e.g., staphylococcal) infection

Laboratory   HSV-2 isolated; bacterial culture negative

Diagnosis   Recurrent genital herpes

Treatment   Local hygiene

Other   Pain and pruritus resolved after 1 day; healed within 8 days

Comment   Typical recurrent genital herpes; acyclovir optional, as most recurrences heal rapidly; patient had 5 similar episodes over next 2 years

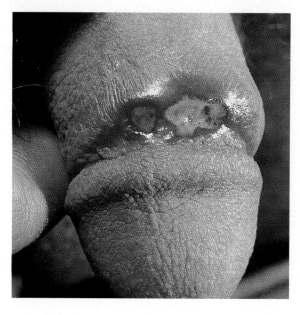

7-3 *Primary genital herpes mimicking chancroid.*

Patient Profile   Age 22, auto mechanic

History   Painful penile sore for 5 days, left groin pain; no systemic symptoms; new sexual partner 10 days earlier

Examination   Tender penile ulcers with purulent bases; no vesicles or pustules; tender, nonfluctuant left inguinal lymphadenopathy with faint overlying erythema

Differential Diagnosis   Herpes, chancroid, syphilis, pyogenic infection

Laboratory   Dark-field examination, syphilis serology, culture for *H. ducreyi* all negative; HSV-1 isolated from lesion

Diagnosis   Genital herpes (due to HSV-1)

Treatment   Acyclovir 400 mg PO TID for 7 days

Other   Clinical appearance suggested chancroid, including warmth and erythema over involved inguinal lymph node; in United States, herpes is the most common cause of chancroid-like genital ulcers, except in presence of local chancroid outbreak or exposure; HSV-1 causes 10–15 percent of genital herpes; partner found to have history of recurrent orolabial herpes

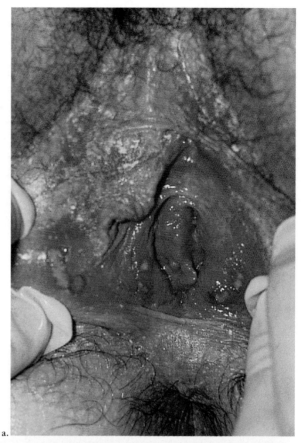

a.

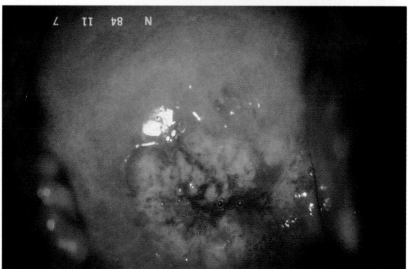

b.

7-4   *Primary genital herpes. a. Multiple introital ulcers b. Ulcerative cervicitis.* (Courtesy of Claire E. Stevens and Lawrence Corey, M.D.)

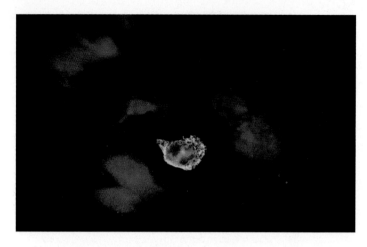

7-5 *Fluorescent antibody stain for HSV-2 in exudate from genital lesion, highlighting an infected cell.* (Courtesy of Syva Corporation, Palo Alto, CA.)

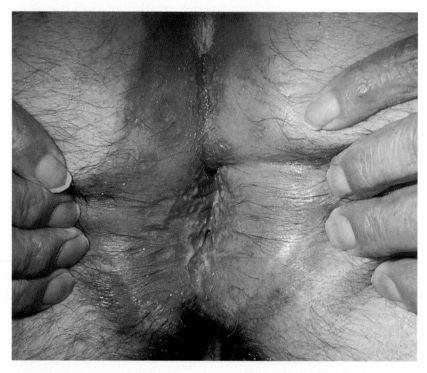

7-6 *Extensive perianal ulcerations due to primary herpes in a homosexual man. The patient also had fever and tenesmus, and anoscopy showed ulcerative proctitis. HSV-2 was isolated.*

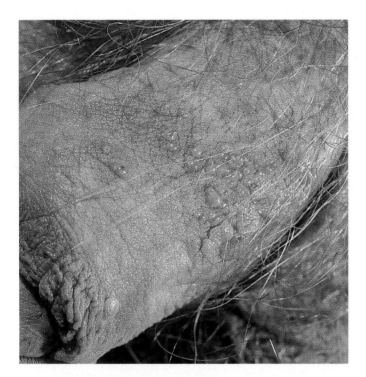

7-7   *Primary genital herpes: extensive vesicular lesions of penis.*

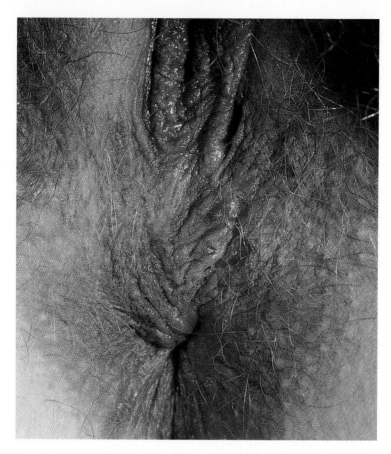

7-8   *Nonprimary first episode genital herpes with unilateral ulcers between introitus and anus. The erythematous lesion adjacent to the anus and the erythema with scale on right side of the perineum are due to psoriasis, which the patient had for several years.*

III   VIRAL SEXUALLY TRANSMITTED DISEASES

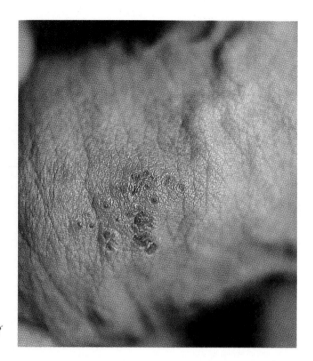

7-9 *Recurrent genital herpes: cluster of crusting lesions on penis.*

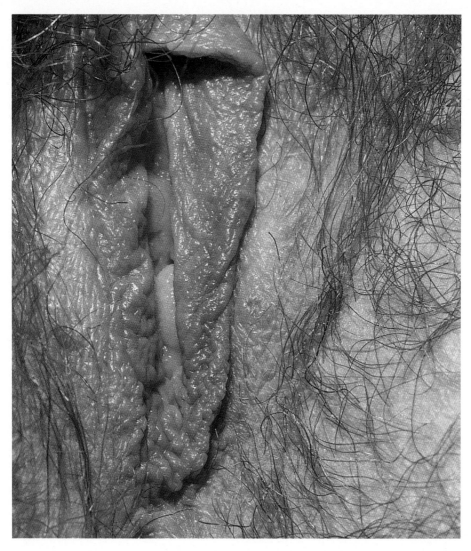

7-10 *Recurrent genital herpes, with a single, 2-mm ulcerative lesion of the labia majora; HSV-2 was isolated from the lesion.*

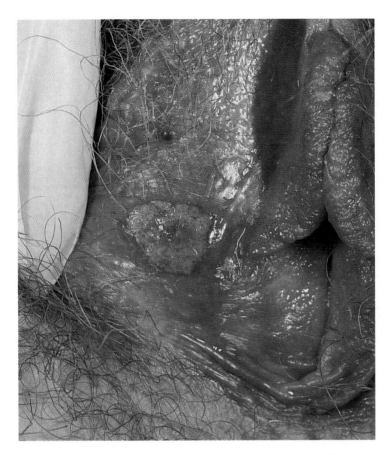

7-11 *Primary genital herpes, with a single, large, ulcerative vulvar lesion mimicking chancroid. (The violaceous lesion anterior to the ulcer is a hemangioma.)*

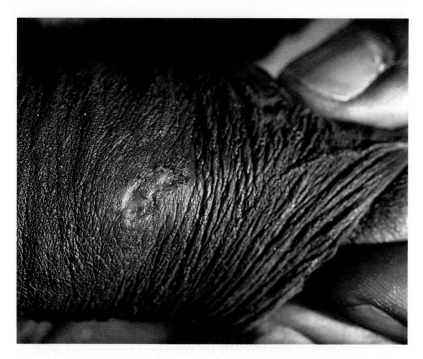

7-12 *Recurrent genital herpes of underside of the penis (note median raphé). Similar lesions, which the patient attributed to catching his penis in his zipper or to other trauma, had occurred periodically for 2 years. HSV-2 was isolated. Some patients with recurrent genital lesions may give assumed but undocumented explanations.*

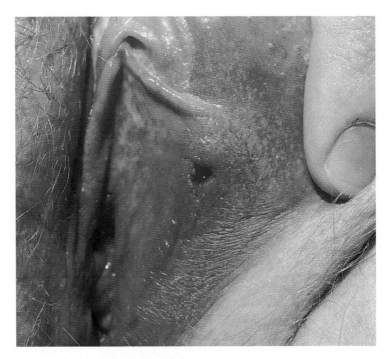

7-13 *Subclinical recurrent genital herpes. The patient sought care because of sexual exposure to gonorrhea and had no complaints referable to the ulcerative lesion. HSV-2 was isolated. In retrospect, she recalled feeling a painless "bump" at the same site several times in the preceding year—an example of subclinical but not truly asymptomatic recurrent outbreaks.*

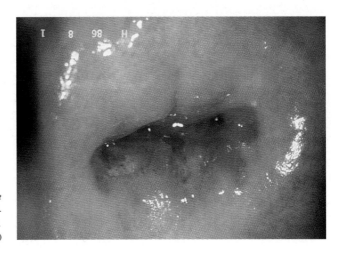

7-14 *Asymptomatic recurrent genital herpes: culture-positive ulcerative lesions in cervical os.* (Courtesy of Claire E. Stevens.)

ADDITIONAL READING

Corey L: Genital herpes, in *Sexually Transmitted Diseases*, 2d ed, KK Holmes et al (eds). New York, McGraw-Hill, 1990, chap 35.

Corey L, Spear PG: Infections with herpes simplex viruses. *N Engl J Med* 314:686, 749, 1986.

Corey L et al: Genital herpes simplex virus infection: Clinical manifestations, course, and complications. *Ann Intern Med* 98:958, 1983.

Kaplowitz LG et al: Prolonged continuous acyclovir treatment of normal adults with frequently recurring genital herpes simplex virus infection. *JAMA* 265:747, 1991.

Koutsky LA et al: The frequency of unrecognized type 2 herpes simplex virus infection among women: Implications for the control of genital herpes. *Sex Transm Dis* 17:90, 1990.

Stone KM, Whittington WL: Treatment of genital herpes. *Rev Infect Dis* 12(suppl 6):S610, 1990.

Chapter 8 Genital Warts and Human Papillomavirus Infection

Genital warts (condylomata acuminata) and infection with human papillomavirus (HPV), long considered an inconvenient but benign condition, has emerged as one of the most common and important STDs. Patients with subclinical HPV infections substantially outnumber those with recognized warts, and in individual patients the cutaneous and mucosal involvement usually is of far greater extent than the visible condylomata. Some HPV strains, especially types 16, 18, and 31, are strongly associated with dysplasia and squamous cell cancer of the cervix, penis, anus, and vulva. Because no treatment has been shown to eradicate the virus, the primary management goals for HPV infection are ablation of exophytic warts, surveillance for malignancy and premalignant changes, and curtailment of transmission through counseling.

EPIDEMIOLOGY

Incidence and Prevalence Estimated >1.2 million annual patient visits to physicians for genital warts in the United States; genital warts are among the most common disorders in STD clinics (typically 10–20 percent of patients); HPV DNA can be detected in the cervix or vulva of 40–70 percent of women attending STD clinics

Transmission Transmitted sexually; perinatally to infants born to infected mothers; autoinoculation from nongenital sites probably is rare

Age No clear predilection; overt genital warts most common in younger sexually active persons, perhaps due to later immunity

Sex No predilection known

Race No known predilection; reflects sexual behaviors

Sexual Orientation Anal and rectal warts common in homosexually active men, possibly related to increased risk of anal squamous cell carcinoma

Other Risk Factors Cellular immunodeficiency (e.g., due to HIV infection) is associated with recrudescence of warts

HISTORY

Incubation Period Warts commonly appear 1–3 months after exposure, but often longer; most infections remain subclinical

Symptoms Visible warts are most common complaint; traumatized warts may be painful or ulcerated; urethral warts in men may cause altered urine stream and rarely outflow obstruction; anecdotal reports suggest association of HPV or warts with some cases of vaginal discharge or vulvar pruritus

Epidemiologic History Often associated with obvious behavioral STD risks, but these may be absent when warts appear

PHYSICAL EXAMINATION

Exophytic warts usually have typical "cauliflower" appearance, but sessile or otherwise atypical warts are common; on mucosal surfaces, magnification of new warts usually reveals frondlike appendages with central capillary; otherwise invisible "flat warts" sometimes can be visualized by application of 3% acetic acid, resulting in "acetowhite" opacification; examination may be entirely normal, with infection revealed only by cytology, biopsy, or detection of HPV DNA; colposcopy useful in women with cervical warts to identify extent of involvement or to guide biopsy

LABORATORY DIAGNOSIS

Typical changes may be seen on Papanicolaou stain of cytologic specimens from cervix, anus, occasionally other sites; biopsy with histologic examination commonly considered definitive, but probably insensitive; tests to detect HPV DNA appear sensitive, but role in routine screening is unknown; annual cervical cytology is indicated for all women with genital warts or sexually exposed to infected partner

DIAGNOSTIC CRITERIA

Visual diagnosis adequate for most cases of exophytic warts; documentation by cytology, histology, or DNA detection usually reliable in experienced laboratory, but negative tests do not reliably exclude infection

TREATMENT

Principles Primary therapy is direct ablation of visible warts; widespread genital skin and mucosal destruction (e.g., laser coagulation) usually is unsuccessful in eradicating HPV and has not been shown to reduce risk of neoplasia or sexual transmission; most modalities require repeated treatment, usually one to three times weekly for 2–6 weeks; patients with warts involving the cervix should be referred to an expert for management

Treatment of Choice For exophytic warts, cryotherapy with liquid nitrogen (using commercial spray device) or cryoprobe; cryoprobe should not be used for intravaginal lesions (risk of fistula formation)

Alternative Regimens Most less effective or less well tolerated than cryotherapy

- Podophyllin resin, 10–25% in compound tincture of benzoin, or 10% purified podophyllotoxin, applied to visible warts and washed off after 2–4 hours; may be increased to 8–24 hours if shorter exposure does not cause severe inflammation
- Trichloroacetic acid, 90% solution
- Interferon-α, injected into base of wart; poorly tolerated and lacking clear advantages over other, less expensive modalities; topical interferon not effective
- Carbon dioxide laser or surgical excision are options for very extensive warts and those that do not respond to nonsurgical therapy

CONTROL MEASURES

Ablation of overt warts presumably reduces viral load and therefore transmissibility; counsel patients to defer sexual contact in presence of visible warts; condoms may prevent transmission of some cases; sexual partners should be examined, but in absence of visible warts special diagnostic methods (colposcopy, application of acetic acid, blind HPV DNA tests, biopsy) are of uncertain utility; screen all patients for syphilis, gonorrhea, and chlamydial infection; counsel about HIV and offer HIV antibody testing

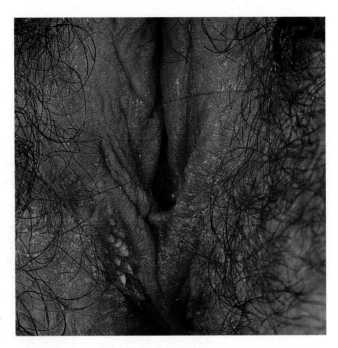

8-1 *Genital warts (condylomata acuminata) of vulva and perineum.*

Patient Profile Age 23, single graduate student

History Painless genital "bumps" for 1 month; monogamous in a relationship that began 4 months earlier

Examination Several warts of labia major and perineum

Diagnosis Genital warts

Laboratory Routine screening for other STD, including VDRL and HIV serology; Pap smear

Treatment Lesions frozen with liquid nitrogen spray; repeat treatments scheduled weekly until resolved

Management of Partner Advised to come for examination for genital warts

Other Patient counseled about potential for recurrence and need for annual Pap smear

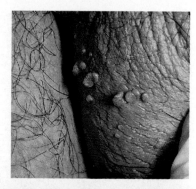

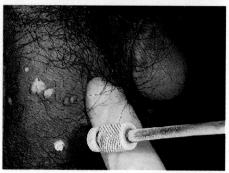

8-2   a. Genital warts of scrotum. b. Same lesions, being frozen with liquid nitrogen spray.

Patient Profile   Age 30, single male assembly line worker

History   Painless scrotal lesions for 2 weeks; three sex partners in past 2 months

Examination   Several 1- to 4-mm warts of scrotum, some cauliflower-like, others smooth

Differential Diagnosis   Genital warts, molluscum contagiosum, secondary syphilis (condylomata lata), nonpigmented nevi

Laboratory   Screening for other STDs, including stat syphilis serology (negative)

Diagnosis   Genital warts

Treatment   Lesions frozen with liquid nitrogen; repeat treatments scheduled weekly until resolved

Other   Counseled about sexually transmitted nature of genital warts; advised to refer partners for evaluation and to use condoms for nonmonogamous sexual encounters

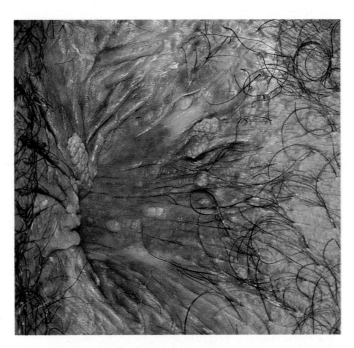

8-3 *Perianal condylomata acuminata.*

Patient Profile   Age 43, homosexual male television cameraman

History   Perianal bumps and itching for 1 week; history of anal warts that resolved with podophyllin therapy 6 years earlier; documented HIV-positive 2 years earlier, with no subsequent follow-up; monogamous for 2 years, with no receptive anal intercourse; no constitutional symptoms

Examination   Numerous perianal excrescences; anoscopy normal, without mucosal warts or lesions; nontender 1- to 2-cm lymph nodes palpable in posterior cervical chain, axillae, and inguinal regions

Differential Diagnosis   Anal warts, syphilis (condylomata lata), carcinoma

Laboratory   VDRL and rectal cultures for *N. gonorrhoeae* and *C. trachomatis* (all negative)

Diagnosis   Anal warts; HIV infection with generalized lymphadenopathy (CDC stage III)

Treatment   Lesions frozen with liquid nitrogen; scheduled for weekly treatments and reexamination (including repeat anoscopy)

Other Advised that recrudescence of warts may be due to advancing immunodeficiency, especially in absence of apparent reexposure; scheduled for follow-up for AIDS-related evaluation (see Chap. 10); warned that warts may be especially difficult to eradicate in presence of HIV infection; if not substantially improved after two or three treatments, referral may be warranted for biopsy (to exclude carcinoma) and surgical extirpation

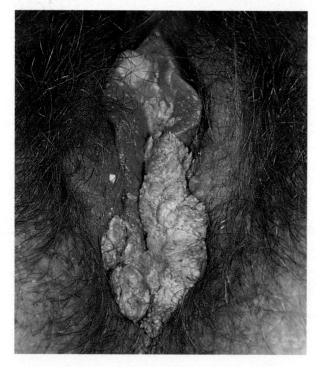

8-4 *Giant condylomata of vulva. Secondary infection and necrosis are common complications of giant warts.*

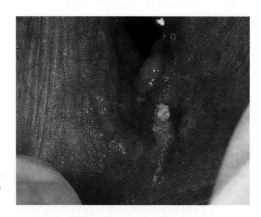

8-5 *Condylomata acuminata of posterior vaginal introitus. On close inspection, central venules can be seen in individual fronds.*

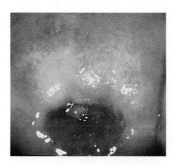 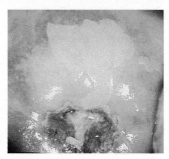

8-6 *Cervix with subclinical "flat" condyloma due to HPV. a. Normal-appearing ectocervix. (Note mucopurulent exudate in os, unrelated to HPV infection; C. trachomatis was isolated.) b. "Acetowhite" flat condyloma revealed by application of 3% acetic acid, viewed in green light. Note that the acetowhite lesion does not correspond to the relatively pale area in a.* (Courtesy of Claire E. Stevens.)

ADDITIONAL READING

Kirby P, Corey L: Genital human papillomavirus infections. *Infect Dis Clin North Am* 1:123, 1987.

Koutsky LA et al: Epidemiology of human papillomavirus infection. *Epidemiol Rev* 10:122, 1988.

Kraus SJ, Stone KM: Management of genital infection caused by human papillomavirus. *Rev Infect Dis* 12(suppl 6):S620, 1990.

Oriel D: Genital human papillomavirus infection, in *Sexually Transmitted Diseases*, 2d ed, KK Holmes et al (eds). New York, McGraw-Hill, 1990, chap 38.

Paavonen J et al: Cervical neoplasia and other STD-related genital and anal neoplasias, in *Sexually Transmitted Diseases*, 2d ed, KK Holmes et al (eds). New York, McGraw-Hill, 1990, chap 48.

Chapter 9   Molluscum Contagiosum

Molluscum contagiosum is a common viral eruption that on cursory examination may resemble genital warts. In sexually active adults, the infection most commonly involves the external genitals, but the most common manifestation overall probably is facial lesions in young children, presumably due to salivary transmission among toddlers. Facial lesions are also common in AIDS patients, suggesting that the molluscum contagiosum virus may persist latently for life and reactivate if immune surveillance fails. Molluscum is a benign condition, with few if any complications except cosmetic ones.

EPIDEMIOLOGY

Incidence and Prevalence   No statistics available; 1–2 percent of diagnoses in STD clinic patients

Transmission   Sexual or salivary transmission

Age   Young children (facial lesions) and sexually active persons (genital lesions)

Sex, Race, Sexual Orientation   No known predisposition

Other Risk Factors   Cellular immunodeficiency is associated with recrudescent lesions

HISTORY

Incubation Period   Probably 1–2 months

Symptoms   Painless papules; often asymptomatic

Epidemiologic History   STD behavioral risks; sometimes contact with known case

PHYSICAL EXAMINATION

Lesions usually have smooth, waxy appearance, often with central umbilication; may superficially resemble warts; atypical appearances occasionally seen; in addition to external genitals, lesions common in pubic area, low abdomen, thighs; facial lesions in adults suggest cellular immune deficiency, such as advanced HIV infection

LABORATORY DIAGNOSIS

No specific tests; characteristic histology if lesion biopsied

DIAGNOSTIC CRITERIA

Clinical appearance; may be confused with genital warts on cursory examination; examine small lesions with magnifying lens; expression of hard, white core confirms diagnosis (commonly followed by brisk bleeding)

TREATMENT

Treatment based on ablation of lesions; freezing with liquid nitrogen or cryoprobe is effective; if few in number, lesions may be unroofed with needle and core manually expressed, although this method carries risks of local reinoculation

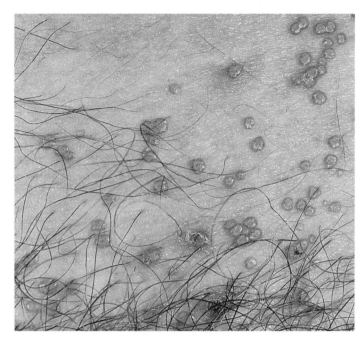

9-1 *Molluscum conta-giosum.*

Patient Profile   Age 19, male college sophomore

History   Painless "bumps" on lower abdomen and pubic area, first noted 2–3 weeks previously; new girlfriend for 2 months

Examination   Numerous 1- to 3-mm superficial, smooth papules, some with central umbilication

Differential Diagnosis   Molluscum contagiosum, genital warts, syphilis (condylomata lata), other papular eruptions

Laboratory   Screening tests for other STDs, including serologic test for syphilis and HIV testing and counseling

Diagnosis   Molluscum contagiosum

Treatment   One lesion unroofed and core expressed, to confirm diagnosis; remainder frozen with liquid nitrogen

Management of Sex Partner(s)   Refer for examination

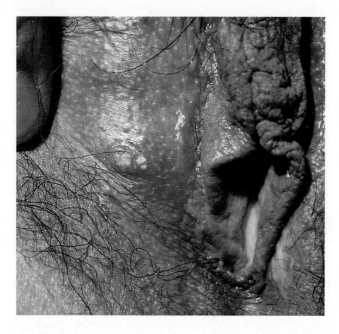

9-2 *Atypical molluscum contagiosum; patient also has discharge
due to bacterial vaginosis.*

Patient Profile   Age 20, single Army-enlisted woman

History   Malodorous vaginal discharge and painless vulvar lesion 1 week; monogamous for past year, but boyfriend known to have other partners

Examination   4-mm nontender papular lesion of vulva with superficial ulceration and firm, white base; homogeneous, white vaginal discharge

Differential Diagnosis   Syphilis, genital wart, herpes, chancroid, molluscum contagiosum, granuloma inguinale, cancer

Laboratory   Dark-field examination, VDRL, culture for HSV (all negative); on attempt at punch biopsy, hard white core extruded; molluscum contagiosum confirmed histologically; screened for gonorrhea and chlamydial infection (negative)

Diagnosis   Molluscum contagiosum; bacterial vaginosis (see also Fig. 18-4)

Treatment   Frozen with liquid nitrogen after core extruded; bacterial vaginosis treated with metronidazole

Management of Sex Partner   Advised to refer partner for examination

Other   Atypical case; ulcerated molluscum lesions rarely recognized

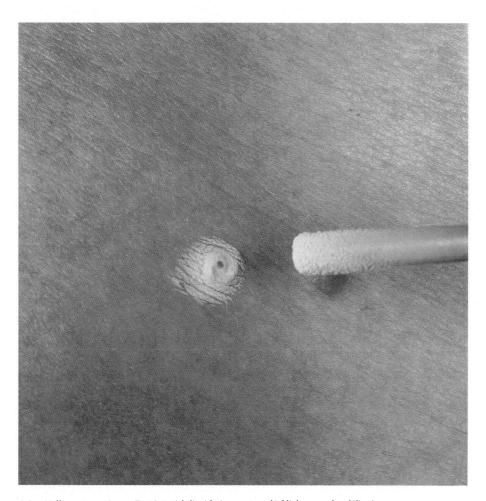

9-3   *Molluscum contagiosum: Freezing with liquid nitrogen spray highlights central umbilication.*

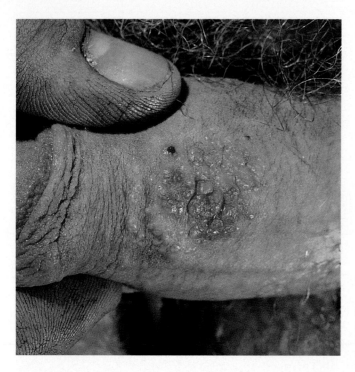

9-4 *Molluscum contagiosum: confluent lesions of penis. Note bleeding after expression of the core of a lesion.*

ADDITIONAL READING

Douglas JM Jr: Molluscum contagiosum, *Sexually Transmitted Diseases,* 2d ed, KK Holmes et al (eds). New York, McGraw-Hill, 1990, chap. 39.

Chapter 10   Human Immunodeficiency Virus Infection

The acquired immunodeficiency syndrome (AIDS) has rapidly become one of history's major public health problems and the most important of all STDs. In all areas of the world, the public health impact of AIDS is amplified by its predominant occurrence in socioeconomically disadvantaged and often stigmatized populations, and the resulting interplay between health care, economics, politics, and social policy currently is more intense than for any other health problem. Worldwide, sexual contact is the predominant route of transmission of the causative agent, human immunodeficiency virus (HIV).

All clinicians who provide care to patients with STD or persons at risk should be prepared to recognize the major signs and symptoms of HIV infection and AIDS, elicit histories of high-risk behavior, provide serologic testing for HIV infection, and educate and counsel patients to reduce their risk of exposure or transmission. It is beyond the scope of this book to review all aspects of HIV infection. Rather, the focus is on the epidemiology of AIDS and HIV infection in the United States, prevention, and the clinical recognition and management of early HIV infection.

EPIDEMIOLOGY

Incidence   Through 1990, 161,073 cases of AIDS reported in the United States; CDC estimates national incidence as 40,000 new HIV infections per year

Prevalence   As of 1990, 0.8–1.2 million persons in the United States estimated to be infected with HIV; 20–40 percent of urban homosexually active men; great geographic variation among intravenous drug users (IVDU), ranging from >60 percent in some eastern cities to <5 percent elsewhere; 0.10–0.15 percent of military recruits; ≤0.01 percent of volunteer blood donors (known high-risk persons excluded); 0.5–3.0 percent of hospital admissions; 0–5 percent of STD clinic patients who deny male homosexuality and IV drug use

Transmission of HIV   Transmitted only by sexual exposure, parenteral contact with infected blood or other body fluids, or perinatally; worldwide, sexual contact is the predominant mode; vaginal or anal intercourse accounts for almost all sexual transmission; transmission by orogenital contact apparently uncommon; kissing probably safe in absence of oral inflammatory lesions or bleeding; factors that contribute to sexual transmission include genital ulcer diseases, perhaps other STD, absence of circumcision, traumatic sexual practices, exposure during menstruation, and advanced immunodeficiency; barrier contraception (e.g., condoms) reduces risk

Age   Distribution reflects peak ages for sexual activity and substance abuse; for overt AIDS, modal age group is 30–39 years and 90 percent are <50 years old

Sex   For overt AIDS, male-female ratio is 9.2:1 overall; 3.4:1 among persons infected by IV drug use; 1:2.4 among those exposed heterosexually

Race Blacks and Hispanics overrepresented relative to their contribution to the population, reflecting racial differences in behavioral risks

Sexual Orientation Homosexual and bisexual men accounted for 59 percent of cumulative reported adult AIDS cases through 1990

Intravenous Drug Use Heterosexual IV drug users accounted for 22 percent of cumulative adult cases through 1990; risk related both to shared injection equipment and sexual exposure

Heterosexual Exposure Through 1990, heterosexual exposure in the United States accounted for 4 percent of cumulative cases overall; 28 percent of cases in women

Other Risk Factors Exposure to infected blood products, donated organs or semen (rare after 1985); perinatal transmission to newborns; breast feeding (rare); occupational exposure of health care workers and laboratory personnel who work with HIV (rare); no documented transmission by arthropods, nonintimate personal exposure (e.g., household contact), or environmental contamination

HISTORY AND CLINICAL MANIFESTATIONS

Epidemiologic History High-risk behavior or exposure since 1977; indirect markers include sexual exposure between men, nonwhite race, residence in high-prevalence geographic areas, illicit drug use, and past or current STD

Incubation Period Seroconversion typically 4–12 weeks after infection, rarely ≥6 months; time from infection to overt AIDS usually is >2 years in adults, with median interval 10–12 years; usually 3 months to 2 years in perinatally exposed infants

Symptoms and Signs Variable, depending on clinical stage (Table 10-1); in STD clinics and similar settings, high proportions of infected persons are asymptomatic or have mild symptoms not obviously related to HIV infection; acute infection may be manifested by mononucleosis-like syndrome, generalized rash, or aseptic meningitis, but most cases asymptomatic; generalized lymphadenopathy; petechiae due to immune thrombocytopenia; manifestations related to increasingly severe immunodeficiency include constitutional symptoms (e.g., fever, weight loss, diarrhea), oropharyngeal signs (e.g., gingivitis, thrush, hairy leukoplakia), cutaneous anomalies (e.g., severe seborrheic dermatitis, telangiectasias of anterior chest, facial warts or molluscum contagiosum, generalized pruritus), neuropsychological manifestations (e.g., memory loss, personality change, dementia, peripheral neuropathy), allergic drug reactions, skin and mucous membrane lesions of Kaposi's sarcoma, and manifestations of opportunistic infection

LABORATORY EVALUATION

Tests for HIV Infection Enzyme-linked immunosorbent assay (ELISA) for HIV antibody, verified by Western blot or other confirmatory test; antibody denotes HIV infection and the potential for transmission, except for some newborns who may remain seropositive for up to 15 months due to transplacental transfer of maternal antibody; false-positive tests for HIV antibody (when verified by confirmatory test) are extremely rare, but indeterminate confirmatory assays remain an occasional problem, especially in persons at low risk; detection of HIV, its antigens, or

Table 10-1
Centers for Disease Control Classification of HIV Infection

GROUP	SYNDROME
I	Acute HIV infection: requires documentation of seroconversion
II	Asymptomatic, seropositive: no current or previous signs or symptoms of infection
III	Persistent generalized lymphadenopathy: palpable lymph nodes at two or more extrainguinal sites
IV	Severe AIDS-related diseases and syndromes
A	Constitutional disease: unexplained fever or diarrhea for more than 1 month or unintentional loss of more than 10% of body weight
B	Neurologic disease: unexplained dementia, myelopathy, or neuropathy
C-1	Opportunistic infection: presence of any of 12 specified systemic or invasive infectious diseases*
C-2	Other infection: oral hairy leukoplakia, multidermatomal herpes zoster, recurrent *Salmonella* bacteremia, nocardiosis, tuberculosis, or oral candidiasis
D	Opportunistic malignancies of the CDC surveillance definition: Kaposi's sarcoma, non-Hodgkin's lymphoma, primary central nervous system lymphoma
E	Other conditions

Pneumocystis carinii pneumonia, chronic cryptosporidiosis, toxoplasmosis, extraintestinal strongyloidiasis, isosporiasis, candidiasis (esophageal, bronchial, or pulmonary), cryptococcosis, histoplasmosis, mycobacterial infection with *Mycobacterium avium* group or *M. kansasii,* symptomatic CMV infection (e.g., retinitis, esophagitis, colitis, pneumonia), chronic mucocutaneous or disseminated HSV infection, and progressive multifocal leukoencephalopathy.

genetic sequences occasionally useful but are primarily research tools

Assessment of Immunologic Function Primary test is quantitation of lymphocyte subsets; normal CD4+ (T4, "helper") lymphocyte count is >600 per mm^3; <200 per mm^3 denotes severe immunodeficiency

Ancillary Tests Complete blood count, platelet count, syphilis serology, tuberculin test (with controls), chemistry panel, urinalysis; hepatitis B and toxoplasma serology; depending on immune function and clinical status, screening or diagnostic tests for opportunistic diseases may be indicated (e.g., chest x-ray, cultures, biopsies, etc); test for β$_2$-microglobulin believed by some investigators to help in assessing prognosis

TREATMENT

Antiretroviral Cheemotherapy Zidovudine (azidothymidine, AZT) 100 mg PO 5 times daily prolongs survival in patients with stage IV HIV infection; higher doses apparently offer no additional benefit and are substantially more toxic; many authorities recommend zidovudine for all patients with CD4+ lymphocyte counts <500 per mm³; other antiretroviral agents are under development

Prevention of Opportunistic Diseases
If tuberculin-positive without active tuberculosis, give isoniazid 300 mg PO once daily for 1 year; pneumococcal vaccine; *Haemophilus influenzae* vaccine; hepatitis B vaccine (if susceptible); influenza vaccine (repeated annually); prophylaxis against *Pneumocystis carinii* pneumonia if CD4+ lymphocyte count <200 per mm³, or if CD4 cells are <20 percent of circulating lymphocytes: effective regimens include sulfamethoxazole/trimethoprim 800/160 mg PO, either once daily or BID on 3 days each week; or aerosol pentamidine by inhalation, 300 mg every 4 weeks

CONTROL MEASURES

General Principles Education to reduce or eliminate high-risk behaviors, directed both to individuals at risk and the population at large, is the primary control measure, pending development of effective HIV vaccine or chemotherapy to prevent transmission. Measures to prevent nonintimate personal contact of infected persons with others (e.g., quarantine, restriction of employment) are unwarranted.

Serologic Screening Many persons at risk modify high-risk behavior more effectively when personal education is combined with testing for HIV infection; serologic screening, with comprehensive pre- and posttest counseling about HIV risks and prevention, should be routinely recommended to persons with any STD or at risk

Management of Sex Partners All infected persons should be advised to inform their past and present sexual or needle-sharing partners; in some states, the clinician or health officials are required by law to take an active role in identification and referral of exposed partners

Reporting Overt AIDS is reportable in all states; reporting requirements for other stages of HIV infection vary widely, with about half the states now requiring reporting of all HIV-positive persons, either with or without identifying information; clinicians should know and cooperate with local reporting requirements

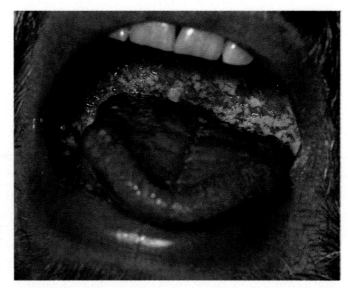

10-1 *Oral candidiasis associated with HIV infection.* (Courtesy of Philip Kirby, M.D.; reprinted with permission from KK Holmes et al, AIDS Dx/Rx. New York, McGraw-Hill, 1990.)

Patient Profile   Age 33, homosexual male flight attendant

History   Intermittent fever for 6 months, 15-pound weight loss; sexual partner recently diagnosed as having AIDS

Examination   Nontender 1- to 2-cm nontender lymph nodes in axillae and posterior cervical chains; prominent seborrheic dermatitis; patchy white exudate of pharynx and buccal mucosa

Laboratory   HIV antibody positive by ELISA, confirmed by Western blot test; VDRL and rectal cultures for *N. gonorrhoeae* and *C. trachomatis* (all negative); hematocrit 41 percent; leukocyte count 5600 per mm^3 with normal differential; CD4+ lymphocytes 326 per mm^3, CD8+ lympocytes 640 per mm^3 (CD4:CD8 ratio 0.51)

Diagnosis   Stage IVA HIV infection with oral candidiasis

Treatment   Zidovudine 100 mg PO 5 times daily (every 4 hours while awake); oral clotrimazole troches for candidiasis

Other   Hepatitis B and toxoplasma serology; tuberculin test with controls; chest x-ray; counseled regarding safe sexual practices and need to refer other past and present sex partners; psychological counseling or referral, if necessary; establish regular follow-up; repeat examination and CD4+ count every 3–6 months; immunizations against *Streptococcus pneumoniae, Haemophilus influenzae* type B, and influenza

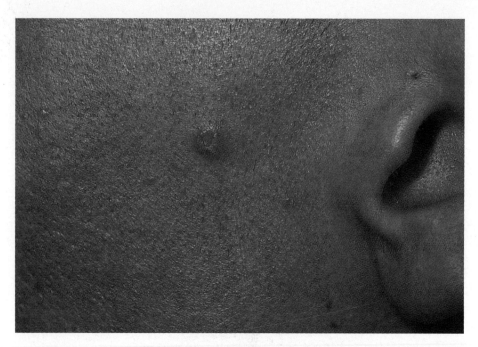

10-2   *Molluscum contagiosum of the cheek in a patient with AIDS. Facial molluscum or warts in adults probably result from recrudescence of latent infection, perhaps dating to childhood, due to cellular immunodeficiency.* (Courtesy of Philip Kirby, M.D.)

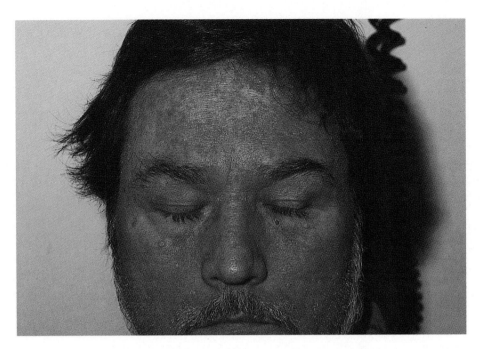

10-3 *Seborrheic dermatitis in AIDS. Severe seborrheic dermatitis is a common manifestation of advanced HIV infection. Note the prominent erythema and fine scale. It usually responds promptly to topical therapy with ketoconazole. The patient also has a molluscum contagiosum lesion below the right eye.* (Courtesy of Philip Kirby, M.D.)

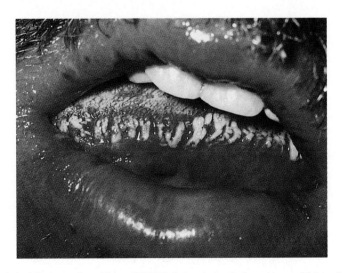

10-4 *Hairy leukoplakia in a patient with stage IV HIV infection. A sign of advanced immunodeficiency, hairy leukoplakia is characterized by painless, hypertrophic, white, vertical striations of the sides of the tongue. Epstein-Barr virus (EBV) has been implicated as a contributing cause. Candida infections can assume a similar appearance. Lesions often regress on oral acyclovir, which has activity against EBV.* (Courtesy of Philip Kirby, M.D.; reprinted with permission from KK Holmes et al (eds), Sexually Transmitted Diseases, 2d ed. New York, McGraw-Hill, 1990.)

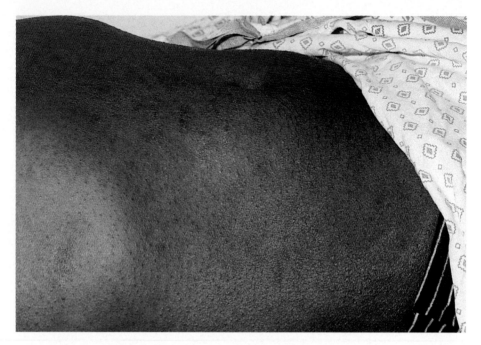

10-5 *AIDS-related icthyosis. HIV-infected persons with advanced immunodeficiency often complain of dry skin and generalized pruritus. The skin feels dry and raspy and a fine scale is present; hyperpigmentation is common. Moisturizing creams are often helpful.* (Courtesy of Philip Kirby, M.D.)

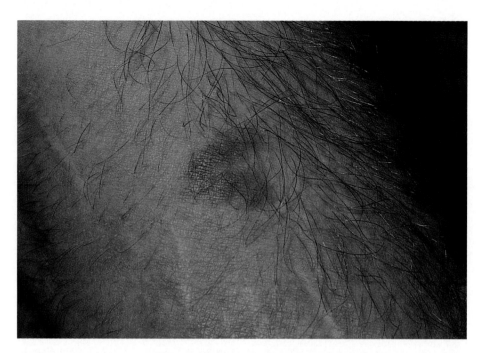

10-6 *Kaposi's sarcoma in AIDS. Most lesions are violaceous or brown nodules, due to vascular proliferation and hemosiderin deposition, but the appearance is highly variable. The diagnosis should be confirmed by biopsy.* (Courtesy of Philip Kirby, M.D.)

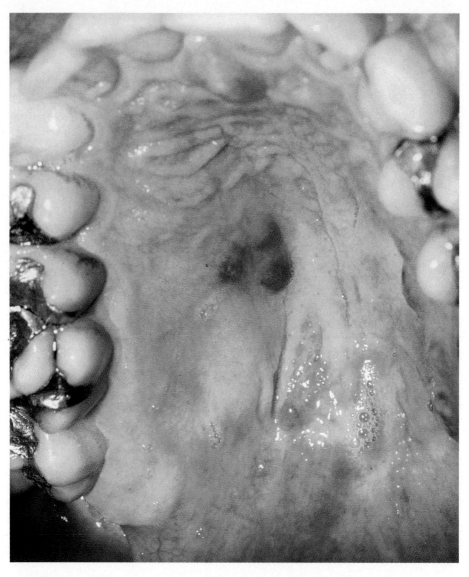

10-7 *Kaposi's sarcoma of the palate in AIDS. Kaposi's sarcoma often presents with oral mucosal lesions.* (Courtesy of James P. Harnisch, M.D.)

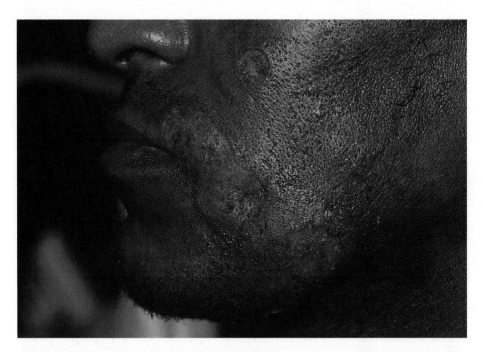

10-8 *Chronic perioral herpes in AIDS. The lesions healed completely on oral acyclovir therapy, which was maintained indefinitely to prevent recurrence.* (Courtesy of Philip Kirby, M.D.)

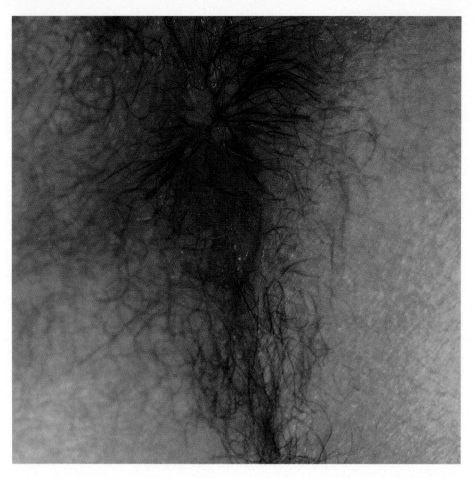

10-9   *Chronic perianal herpes in an HIV-infected patient. Such lesions are extremely painful and often debilitating but respond to oral acyclovir.*

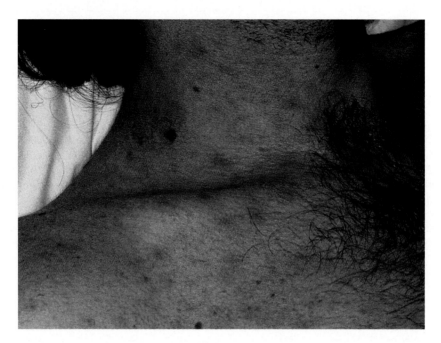

10-10 *Primary HIV infection. There are numerous poorly demarcated erythematous macules and papules of the neck and upper trunk. The patient also had a mononucleosis-like syndrome with fever, pharyngitis, and generalized lymphadenopathy. He was HIV-seronegative, but HIV p24 antigen was detected and HIV antibody developed after 4 weeks.* (Courtesy of David Spach, M.D. and Philip Kirby, M.D.)

ADDITIONAL READING

Brookmeyer R: Reconstruction and future trends of the AIDS epidemic in the United States. *Science* 253:37, 1991.

Cates W Jr, Handsfield HH: Does testing and counseling reduce HIV transmission? editorial. *Am J Public health* 78:1533, 1988.

Curran JW et al: Epidemiology of HIV infection and AIDS in the United States. *Science* 239:610, 1988.

Holmes KK et al (eds): *AIDS Dx/Rx.* New York, McGraw-Hill, 1990.

Holmes KK et al: The increasing frequency of heterosexually acquired AIDS in the United States, 1983–1988. *Am J Public Health* 80:858, 1990.

Chapter 11   Hepatitis B, Cytomegalovirus, and Other Viruses

Hepatitis B virus (HBV) and cytomegalovirus (CMV), like HIV, are carried in the blood and genital secretions and are transmitted by blood contact, exchange of genital secretions, and perinatally. CMV also is transmitted through saliva. Hepatitis C virus (HCV), Epstein-Barr virus (EBV), human T lymphotropic virus types 1 and 2 (HTLV-1 and -2), and perhaps other agents probably share the same transmission characteristics and epidemiology. All of these viruses cause primary infections that are usually asymptomatic, followed by chronic or latent infection with the potential for complications months or years after acquisition. Hepatitis D virus (HDV; formerly "delta agent") is an "incomplete" virus that causes disease only in the presence of HBV infection, resulting in clinical exacerbations and an increased risk of chronic hepatitis and cirrhosis. Hepatitis A virus (HAV) can also be transmitted sexually but is not known to cause chronic infection or late complications. Although not considered STDs, it is likely that most enteric viruses can be transmitted sexually as well.

In addition to acute and chronic hepatitis, chronic HBV infection is closely linked to hepatocellular carcinoma, the most common fatal malignancy in many developing countries. Sexually transmitted hepatitis B was an extremely common problem among homosexually active men in industrialized countries until the mid-1980s. Currently about 25 percent of cases in adults are attributed to heterosexual transmission, 30 percent to sharing of injection equipment among IV drug users, and 5–10 percent to male homosexual transmission; the route of acquisition is unknown in 35–40 percent. HBV is the only sexually transmitted pathogen for which immunization is available. Vaccination programs have been inhibited by the high cost of the vaccine and logistical considerations, including difficulty in reaching the populations at highest risk and the requirement for 3 doses of vaccine over 6 months. Homosexually active men, IV drug users, their sexual partners, and other persons with STD or at risk should be offered HBV vaccination, usually preceded by serologic testing to determine HBV infection status.

Sexual transmission has been documented as an important mode of acquisition of CMV in some demographic settings. Among CMV-seronegative women attending STD clinics, the incidence of primary infection is 8–30 percent per year. Although primary infection in adults is almost always asymptomatic, transmission in utero or perinatally is common. CMV is a major cause of congenital neurodevelopmental abnormalities in the United States. Most congenital or perinatal infections occur in children born to chronically infected mothers, but the risk of clinically significant congenital infection is highest when primary CMV infection occurs in pregnancy. Life-threatening recrudescence of chronic CMV infection is common in AIDS patients and usually presents as pneumonia, retinitis, esophagitis, or colitis. The antiviral drug ganciclovir offers the prospect of partial control of these conditions, if not cure. Routine screening or diagnosis of CMV infection is rarely warranted in adults in the absence of settings that suggest opportunistic CMV disease. Pending development of a safe and effective vaccine, efforts at prevention and control of sexually transmitted CMV probably are not warranted.

ADDITIONAL READING

Alter MJ et al: The changing epidemiology of hepatitis B in the United States: Need for alternative vaccination strategies. *JAMA* 263:1218, 1990.

Collier AC et al: Cytomegalovirus infection in women attending a sexually transmitted disease clinic. *J Infect Dis* 162:46, 1990.

Lemon SM, Newbold JE: Viral hepatitis, in *Sexually Transmitted Diseases,* 2d ed, KK Holmes et al (eds). New York, McGraw-Hill, 1990, chap 40.

Smiley L, Huang E-S: Cytomegalovirus as a sexually transmitted infection, in *Sexually Transmitted Diseases,* 2d ed, KK Holmes et al (eds). New York, McGraw-Hill, 1990, chap 36.

Cutaneous Infestations

Chapter 12 Pediculosis Pubis

Pediculosis pubis, infestation with the crab louse (*Phthirus pubis*), is often sexually acquired, but exceptions are common. Complications are rare, and infestation is more a nuisance than a significant threat to health. Pediculosis pubis is a marker of STD risk, and infested persons should be routinely screened for other STDs.

EPIDEMIOLOGY

Incidence and Prevalence Very common, but no reliable statistics available; diagnosed in 2–4 percent of patients attending STD clinics

Transmission Usually requires pubic apposition, because the crab louse is slowly mobile and does not survive in clothing or fomites; however, exceptions apparently are common

Age Reflects sexual behavioral risks

Sex No special predilection

Race Common in all races

Sexual Orientation No special predilection

Other Risk Factors Communal living (e.g., shelters for homeless persons)

HISTORY

Incubation Period Ova (nits) hatch in 5–10 days; hatched nymphs mature 6–9 days later and begin laying nits

Symptoms Visible nits or lice often are the only complaint; sometimes pruritus

Epidemiologic History Behavioral risks for STD; sexual contact with known case; communal living

PHYSICAL EXAMINATION

Nits, attached at base of hair, are the most common and often only sign of infestation; lice often difficult to find; usually limited to pubic area, but can extend to thighs, trunk; eyelashes occasionally involved, scalp almost never; hemorrhagic macules (maculae ceruleae) at site of feeding are pathognomonic but uncommon

LABORATORY DIAGNOSIS

If diagnosis in doubt on visual inspection, characteristic nits and lice may be examined microscopically

DIAGNOSTIC CRITERIA

Identification of nits, lice, or maculae ceruleae

TREATMENT

Lindane (gamma benzene hexachloride) shampoo or lotion, pyrethrin lotion, or permethrin 1% cream; applied to pubic area, intergluteal fold, from knees to waist, and to any other visibly infested areas (except eyelashes); apply petroleum jelly to infested eyelashes; no treatment reliably kills nits, and reapplication after 5–7 days is recommended to kill hatchlings before maturity

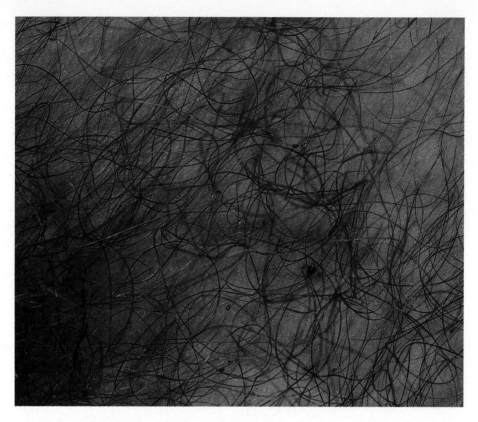

12-1 *Crab louse infestation. Note louse and several nits attached to pubic hairs.*

Patient Profile   Age 33, male construction worker

History   Pubic area itching for 1 week; saw "white things" in pubic hair 1 day earlier; occasional casual sexual contacts

Examination   Nits and typical crab lice in public hair; otherwise normal

Diagnosis   Pediculosis pubis

Treatment   Lindane shampoo; repeated in 7 days

Management of Sex Partner(s)   Advised to inform partners

Other   Screen for HIV and other STDs

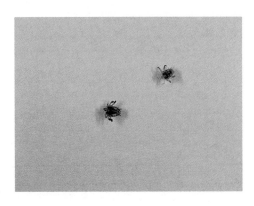

12-2   Phthirus pubis.

ADDITIONAL READING

Billstein SA: Human lice, in *Sexually Transmitted Diseases,* 2d ed, KK Holmes et al (eds). New York, McGraw-Hill, 1990, chap 41.

Chapter 13 Scabies

Scabies is cutaneous infestation with the itch mite, *Sarcoptes scabei.* The organism is transmitted by skin-to-skin contact, and sexual exposure is a common but not exclusive mode of transmission. Scabies is among the most common dermatoses in patients at risk for STD, partly because genital lesions are common. The primary clinical manifestation is an intensely pruritic papular eruption, mediated by hypersensitivity to the burrowing mite and its feces and ova. Scabies often is complicated by secondary staphylococcal or streptococcal infection.

EPIDEMIOLOGY

Incidence and Prevalence No accurate incidence data; accounts for up to 5 percent of STD clinic patients

Transmission Skin-to-skin contact; sexual exposure is a common mode in young adults

Age All ages affected; most common in young children (through nonsexual exposure) and young adults

Race, Gender, Sexual Orientation No special predilection

HISTORY

Incubation Period Typically 2–4 weeks for first episode; often <24 hours for recurrent scabies, due to hypersensitivity resulting from prior infestation

Symptoms Localized or generalized rash with intense pruritus, often worse at night; absence of pruritus is evidence against scabies

Epidemiologic History At risk for STD; communal living; history of exposure

PHYSICAL EXAMINATION

Papular rash, occasionally with 0.5- to 1.0-cm linear lesions ("burrows") that mark the paths of migrating mites; occasional vesicular or nodular lesions; excoriations, eczematous plaques, and secondarily infected lesions (pustules, localized cellulitis) are common; most prominent locations are axillae, flexor surfaces of elbows, hands (especially finger webs), waist, ankles, dorsal surfaces of feet, genitals, buttocks, inguinal and gluteal folds

LABORATORY DIAGNOSIS

Scrapings of lesions examined microscopically in mineral oil or 10% KOH solution often reveal mite, ova, or fecal pellets; biopsy occasionally useful to document atypical cases

DIAGNOSTIC CRITERIA

Diagnosis is based primarily on clinical criteria; application of water-based ink may highlight burrows ("burrow ink test"); microscopic confirmation should be attempted, especially for atypical cases; response to treatment often helpful (therapeutic trial)

TREATMENT

Principles Single application of scabicide usually sufficient, but some authorities routinely re-treat 7 days later; pruritus and lesions may persist 2 weeks or longer, due to hypersensitivity to mites and detritus; treat sexual partners and other close personal contacts

Treatment of Choice Permethrin 5% cream applied to entire skin surface and washed off after 1–2 hours

Alternative Regimens Lindane 1% lotion has efficacy similar to permethrin, but contraindicated in pregnancy and potentially toxic in children; crotamiton is less effective; sulfur in petrolatum is effective but aesthetically unacceptable to most patients

Ancillary Measures Launder bed linens and clothing worn within 48 hours prior to treatment

Management of Sex Partners Routine examination and treatment for sexual contacts and persons who share the patient's living quarters

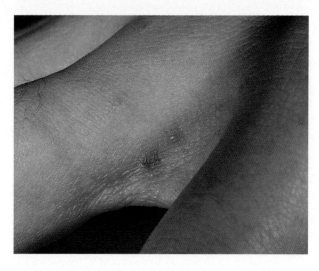

13-1 *Scabies papules of finger web.*

Patient Profile   Age 19, male carpenter

History   Itching "all over" for 2 weeks, worse at night

Examination   Erythematous papules and excoriations of hands, elbows, around waist

Differential Diagnosis   Scabies, eczema, dermatitis herpetiformis, contact dermatitis

Laboratory   Microscopic examination of lesion scrapings demonstrated mite, ova, and feces

Diagnosis   Scabies

Treatment   Permethrin 5% cream; counseled to launder bed linens and clothing used in preceding 48 hours

Management of sex partner(s)   Arrange for examination and treatment

Other   Screen for other STDs

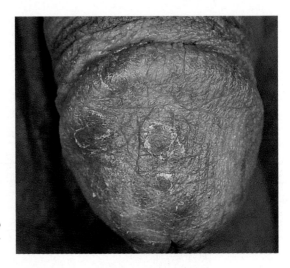

13-2 *Scabies of penis. Note similarity to secondary syphilis and psoriasis (Figs. 4-12, 21-3, 21-4).*

Patient Profile　Age 37, unemployed homeless man living in communal shelter

History　Pruritic rash for 4 weeks, worse at night; no recent sexual exposure

Examination　Hyperkeratotic penile papules; numerous nonspecific papules, nodules, excoriations of trunk (not shown)

Differential Diagnosis　Keratoderma blenorrhagica (Reiter's syndrome), secondary syphilis, psoriasis, eczema, etc.

Laboratory　Patient refused to permit scraping of lesions

Diagnosis　Probable scabies

Treatment　Lindane, 1% lotion

Other　Shelter manager advised to launder patient's linens and clothes, and to refer other residents who have compatible symptoms

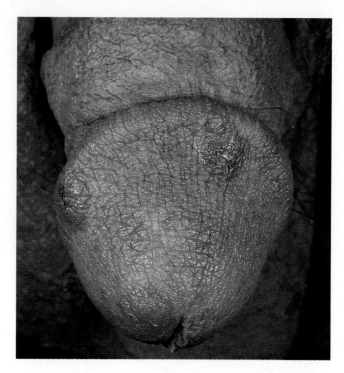

13-3   *Penile scabies. Note absence of scales (compare with Fig. 13-2).*

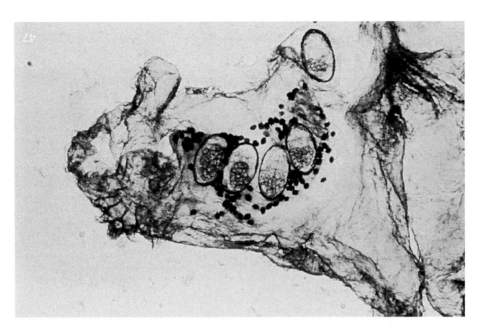

13-4 *Photomicrograph of scraping of fresh scabies papule, showing an intact mite, several ova, and fecal pellets.* (Courtesy of the American Academy of Dermatology Teaching Collection.)

ADDITIONAL READING

Orkin M, Maibach H: Scabies, in *Sexually Transmitted Diseases,* 2d ed, KK Holmes et al (eds). New York, McGraw-Hill, 1990, chap 42.

Schultz MW et al: Comparative study of permethrin 5% cream and lindane 1% lotion for treatment of scabies. *Arch Dermatol* 126:167, 1990.

Clinical STD Syndromes

Chapter 14   Nongonococcal Urethritis

Nongonococcal urethritis (NGU), by definition, is acute urethritis not due to *Neisseria gonorrhoeae,* and is the most common clinical disorder among men presenting to most STD clinics. The term "nonspecific" urethritis is discouraged, because it fosters the notion that the cause is unknown or unknowable. About 30–50 percent of cases are due to *Chlamydia trachomatis* and 20–30 percent probably are caused by the genital mycoplasma *Ureaplasma urealyticum.* Some cases may be caused by the newly described *Mycoplasma genitalium.* A few cases are due to *Trichomonas vaginalis* or HSV (usually with overt penile herpetic lesions), but the etiology is unknown in up to one-third of cases. Coliform bacteria occasionally cause urethritis following insertive anal intercourse. Persisting beliefs that altered frequency of sexual behavior, alcohol, highly spiced foods, physical "strain," and similar factors cause NGU are without basis in fact. However, it remains possible that noninfectious immunologic factors may cause some cases. For example, NGU often accompanies Reiter's syndrome triggered by enteric infection in sexually inactive persons. Postgonococcal urethritis is NGU that follows gonorrhea when dual infection is present and treatment is active only against *N. gonorrhoeae.* The major complications of NGU are acute epididymitis and Reiter's syndrome, which occur primarily in association with *C. trachomatis.* However, these are relatively uncommon, and the major significance of NGU is that it denotes the potential for serious complications in the patients' female sexual partners.

EPIDEMIOLOGY

Incidence and Prevalence   Accurate data unavailable; present in 20–30 percent of men in some STD clinics (two to three times as common as gonorrhea); up to 10 times more common than gonorrhea in patients attending most physicians' offices

Transmission   Initial episodes almost always acquired sexually; some cases of recurrent nonchlamydial NGU are due to relapse of prior infection

Age   Most cases age 15–35; all ages susceptible

Sex   By definition, NGU occurs only in men; female counterpart is mucopurulent cervicitis (see Chap. 17)

Race   No specific predilection

Sexual Orientation   Occurs in both heterosexual and homosexually active men; in the latter, *C. trachomatis* accounts for ≤10 percent of cases and risk of coliform infection increased

HISTORY

Incubation Period   Typically 1–3 weeks, sometimes longer; prolonged asymptomatic infection common

Symptoms   Primarily urethral discharge; dysuria usually mild, often absent; urethral pruritus; severe dysuria with scant discharge suggests herpes

Epidemiologic History History of exposure or high-risk sexual activity, but exceptions common

PHYSICAL EXAMINATION

Urethral discharge, usually mucoid or mucopurulent and less copious than in gonorrhea, but overt purulent exudate sometimes seen; some patients lack demonstrable discharge, depending partly on time since urination; occasional meatal erythema or penile edema

LABORATORY DIAGNOSIS

Gram-Stained Smear Smear of exudate showing ≥5 (usually ≥15) neutrophils per oil immersion (1000×) microscopic field, in an area of the smear that contains a maximum concentration of cellular material; absence of gram-negative diplococci

Microbiologic Tests Collect urethral specimen by passing small swab 2–4 cm into penis for culture or other test for *C. trachomatis;* culture for *N. gonorrhoeae;* cultures for *U. urealyticum* usually not helpful (prevalence of infection is similar in sexually active men with or without urethritis); test for HSV or *T. vaginalis* if indicated by clinical manifestations or exposure history

Other Tests When urethral swab not possible or if smear nondiagnostic despite history suggesting urethritis, obtain first 15–30 ml of voided urine, centrifuge, and examine sediment microscopically for PMNs (≥10 PMNs per 400× field suggests genitourinary inflammation); leukocyte esterase dipstick test on such specimens also may be useful to screen for pyuria due to urethritis; recent studies suggest antigen detection tests for *C. trachomatis* on centrifuged urine sediment

may be useful, but culture of urine is insensitive; obtain VDRL; recommend HIV test

DIAGNOSTIC CRITERIA

Diagnostic criteria in men without evidence of gonorrhea, while awaiting results of tests for *C. trachomatis* and *N. gonorrhoeae:*

1. History of urethral discharge or dysuria
2. Urethral exudate on physical examination
3. Documentation of urethral inflammation by Gram-stained smear showing ≥5 PMNs per 1000× field; or positive leukocyte esterase test on initial 15–30 ml of voided urine

Presence of two or three criteria is presumptively diagnostic of NGU; if only one criterion present, reevaluate after 4–5 days, when patient has not urinated for 4–8 hours (e.g., after overnight retention of urine)

TREATMENT

Treatment of Choice Doxycycline 100 mg PO BID for 7 days

Alternative Regimens Tetracycline HCl 500 mg PO QID for 7 days; erythromycin 2.0 g PO daily in three to four divided doses for 7–10 days; sulfamethoxazole 1.0 g PO BID for 7–10 days, or other sulfonamide in therapeutically equivalent dose (effective for chlamydial infection but not for nonchlamydial NGU); all penicillins and cephalosporins are ineffective; quinolones under investigation (variable results to date)

Recurrent NGU Relapse of urethritis occurs within 6 weeks in 10–20 percent of men with chlamydial NGU and 20–40 percent with nonchlamydial NGU; if no history suggesting reinfection, treat with erythromycin, because some cases may be due to tetracycline-resistant *U. urealyticum;* some authorities empirically treat second recurrences with doxycycline 100 mg PO BID for 3–4 weeks; some recurrences may be due to prostate infection, and some apparent ones may be psychogenic; recurrent symptoms should not be treated with antimicrobial drugs unless there is objective evidence of inflammation

CONTROL MEASURES

As for chlamydial infection and gonorrhea (Chaps. 2 and 3); sexual partners should be examined and treated

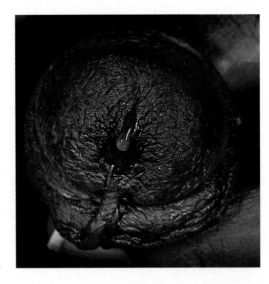

14-1   *Nongonococcal urethritis. See also Fig. 3-1.*

Patient Profile   Age 26, single heterosexual computer programmer

History   Urethral "itching" and intermittent discharge for 7 days; began a new sexual relationship 6 weeks earlier

Examination   Mucopurulent urethral discharge

Differential Diagnosis   NGU, gonorrhea; small likelihood of trichomonal or herpetic urethritis

Laboratory   Urethral Gram stain showed 15–20 PMNs per 1000× field and scant mixed bacterial flora, without gram-negative diplococci; cultured for *C. trachomatis* and *N. gonorrhoeae* (both negative); VDRL and HIV tests (both negative)

Diagnosis   Nongonococcal urethritis

Treatment   Doxycycline 100 mg PO BID for 7 days

Other   Patient counseled about sexually acquired nature of his infection; arrangements made for examination and treatment of partner; follow-up optional if symptoms resolve and partner treated

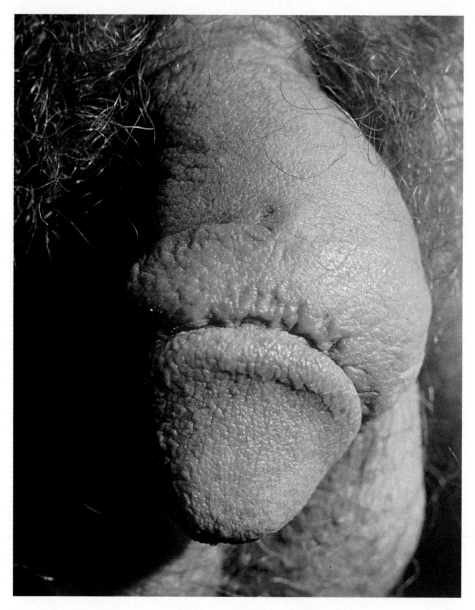

14-2 *"Penile venereal edema" in a patient with chlamydial NGU. Similar to "bull-headed clap" (Fig. 2-7), penile venereal edema is a rare complication of chlamydial infection, gonorrhea, and perhaps nonchlamydial NGU, genital herpes, or other infections. It usually is painless, without tenderness, erythema, or other inflammatory signs, and responds promptly to routine treatment of the underlying infection.*

V   CLINICAL STD SYNDROMES

ADDITIONAL READING

Bowie WR: Urethritis in males, in *Sexually Transmitted Diseases,* 2d ed, KK Holmes et al (eds). New York, McGraw-Hill, 1990, chap 52.

Bowie WR et al: Therapy for nongonococcal urethritis: Double-blind comparison of two doses and two durations of minocycline. *Ann Intern Med* 95:306, 1981.

Hooton TM, Barnes RC: Urethritis in men. *Infect Dis Clin North Am* 1:165, 1987.

Shafer MA et al: Urinary leukocyte esterase screening test for asymptomatic chlamydial and gonococcal infection in males. *JAMA* 262:2562, 1989.

Chapter 15 Epididymitis

As with pelvic inflammatory disease in women, acute epididymitis results from ascending lower genital tract infection. *Chlamydia trachomatis* is the most common cause in sexually active men <35 years old, but some cases are due to *Neisseria gonorrhoeae*. In older men or following urinary tract instrumentation, most cases are due to coliform bacteria, *Pseudomonas*, or other uropathogens.

EPIDEMIOLOGY

Incidence and Prevalence No accurate statistics available; in sexually active men <35 years old, 60–70 percent due to *C. trachomatis*, and about 10 percent due to *N. gonorrhoeae*, depending on local incidences of chlamydia and gonorrhea; estimated to occur in 1–2 percent of men with chlamydial NGU

Transmission As for *C. trachomatis* and *N. gonorrhoeae*

Age Most cases age 15–35

Race No specific predilection

Sexual Orientation No predilection except as related to specific sexual practices; unprotected insertive anal intercourse increases risk of coliform urethritis and epididymitis

Other Risk Factors Urinary tract instrumentation; bacterial prostatitis; anatomic abnormalities that predispose to urinary tract infections in men

HISTORY

Incubation Period Not well studied; usually follows acquisition of urethral chlamydial or gonococcal infection by several days to weeks

Symptoms Testicular pain and swelling, often severe, usually unilateral; sometimes poorly localized (visceral) low abdominal pain; symptoms usually develop over 1–2 days, but some patients report sudden onset; fever may occur but is uncommon; symptoms of urethritis usually mild or absent for chlamydial epididymitis, but typically prominent for gonococcal cases

Epidemiologic History Often high-risk sexual exposure

PHYSICAL EXAMINATION

Epididymal and testicular enlargement, usually with marked tenderness; scrotal erythema often present; signs or laboratory evidence of urethritis usually present, but exceptions are common

LABORATORY DIAGNOSIS

Microscopy Compatible with NGU or gonorrhea (see Chaps. 2, 3, and 14); midstream urine specimen may show coliforms and pyuria

Microbiologic Tests   Urethral cultures for *C. trachomatis* and *N. gonorrhoeae;* midstream urine culture for uropathogens

Other Tests   Midstream urinalysis or leukocyte esterase test to assess pyuria; obtain blood cultures if febrile; stat assessment of blood flow (e.g., Doppler, technetium 99m scan) in patients at risk for testicular torsion, including adolescents, all patients with sudden onset, those without urethritis or pyuria, or if testicle elevated in scrotal sac

DIAGNOSTIC CRITERIA

Epididymal or testicular tenderness and swelling, evidence of urethritis or bacterial urinary tract infection, and absence of alternate diagnoses; differential diagnosis includes "the 4 T's": *T*orsion, *T*umor (i.e., testicular cancer), *T*rauma (usually with history of specific injury), and *T*uberculosis or other granulomatous infections

TREATMENT

Ceftriaxone 250 mg IM plus doxycycline 100 mg PO BID for 10 days is recommended empiric therapy for acute epididymitis in young men, pending results of cultures and susceptibility testing; in older men or following urinary tract instrumentation, give ciprofloxacin 500 mg PO BID (or other fluoroquinolone in equivalent dosage), or other broadspectrum antibiotic therapy

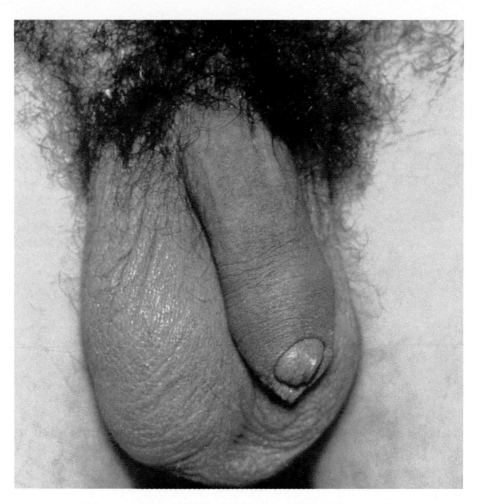

15-1   *Acute epididymitis of right testicle.* (Courtesy of Walter E. Stamm, M.D.)

Patient Profile   Age 28, married electrical engineer

History   Mild right testicular pain beginning 2 days earlier, while playing basketball; pain worse and testicle swollen on awakening the morning of examination; denied urethral discharge and dysuria; sexual intercourse one month previously with a woman he met at party

Examination   Scrotum warm, skin erythematous; testicle indurated, almost twice normal size; marked tenderness, maximal posteriorly, extending into spermatic cord; scant mucoid urethral discharge on "milking" penis

Differential Diagnosis Acute epididymitis; possible trauma, torsion, cancer, granulomatous inflammation

Laboratory Urethral Gram stain showed >15 PMNs per 1000× (oil immersion) microscopic field, without gram-negative diplococci; negative leukocyte esterase test for pyuria on midstream urine sample; urethral cultures sent for *C. trachomatis* (positive) and *N. gonorrhoeae* (negative); midstream urine culture (no growth); VDRL, HIV serology (both negative)

Diagnosis Chlamydial epididymitis

Treatment Ceftriaxone 250 mg IM plus doxycycline 100 mg PO BID for 10 days

Management of Sex Partner(s) Advised to refer wife and new partner for evaluation and treatment for presumptive chlamydia infection

Other Counseled about risks associated with unprotected intercourse with unknown partners; condom use advised

ADDITIONAL READING

Berger RE: Acute epididymitis, in *Sexually Transmitted Diseases,* 2d ed, KK Holmes et al (eds). New York, McGraw-Hill, 1990, chap 53.
Berger RE et al: Etiology and manifestations of epididymitis in young men: Correlation with sexual orientation. *J Infect Dis* 155:1341, 1987.

Chapter 16   Reiter's Syndrome

Reiter's syndrome is classically described as a triad of urogenital inflammation (usually nongonococcal urethritis or cervicitis), seronegative arthritis, and mucocutaneous inflammatory lesions, including conjunctivitis, oral mucosal ulcers, and characteristic dermatitis. However, limited forms of Reiter's syndrome (e.g., "sexually acquired reactive arthritis") are probably more common than the full syndrome. Reiter's syndrome is related to other reactive spondyloarthropathies, such as ankylosing spondylitis, and appears to result from an aberrant immune response following any of several mucosal infections. Anecdotal reports suggest that the incidence of Reiter's syndrome or variants may be increased in patients with HIV infection. From 80–90 percent of affected persons have the histocompatibility locus-A (HLA) B27 tissue haplotype, compared with <10 percent of the general population.

"Epidemic" Reiter's syndrome typically follows shigellosis, yersiniosis, or other enteric infections, whereas the "endemic" form is usually triggered by a genital infection. Overt epidemics have been reported in populations with particularly high prevalences of HLA-B27 positivity, as in Scandinavia. In the United States, genital *C. trachomatis* infection is the most common triggering event. Some evidence suggests that gonorrhea may trigger occasional cases ("postgonococcal arthritis"). Differentiation of Reiter's syndrome from gonococcal arthritis is occasionally difficult, especially in sexually active persons who lack the characteristic skin lesions of either syndrome. Some patients develop permanent disability due to chronic arthritis, but most cases are transient or cause only mild chronic limitations.

EPIDEMIOLOGY

Incidence and Prevalence   Accurate statistics not available; among the most common causes of inflammatory arthritis in sexually active young adults

Transmission   Depends on triggering infection; person-to-person transmission of chlamydia-linked Reiter's syndrome has been documented

Age   Most U.S. cases occur in sexually active age groups; all ages apparently susceptible; epidemics triggered by *Shigella, Yersinia,* or *Campylobacter* have occurred in children as well as adults

Sex   Male-female ratio is 10:1 in some studies, probably due in part to reporting bias or to underdiagnosis of lower genital tract inflammation in women; recent series suggest true male-female ratio is 1:1 to 2:1

Race   Less common in nonwhite populations, probably due to lower prevalence of HLA-B27 haplotype (1–2 percent of blacks, 7–10 percent of whites)

Sexual Orientation   No special predilection; homosexually active men may be at increased risk due to sexually transmitted enteric infections, but no data available

Other Risk Factors   HIV-infected persons appear to be at increased risk and may have more debilitating course

HISTORY

Incubation Period Usually 1–4 weeks after onset of urethritis, cervicitis, or enteric infection

Symptoms Pain, swelling, and limited mobility of any of several joints and tendon insertion sites; usually one to three joints involved in acute episodes; most common sites are heel, toes, lumbosacral spine, knee, or ankle, but any joint can be affected; symptoms of urethritis or cervicitis often present; some patients have recent symptoms of enteric infection; fever and other systemic symptoms usually mild or absent; skin rash and conjunctivitis are variable, sometimes asymptomatic

Epidemiologic History Most cases have behavioral risks for STD; sometimes exposure to enteric infection, occasionally in association with epidemic outbreaks of shigellosis, yersiniosis, or *Campylobacter* infection

PHYSICAL EXAMINATION

Triggering Infection Characteristic signs of NGU, mucopurulent cervicitis, or enteric infection (see Chaps. 14, 17, 20); rarely gonorrhea

Arthropathy Inflammatory signs of one or more joints or tendon insertion sites; diffuse synovitis of one or more toes ("sausage toe") is uncommon but pathognomonic; effusions usually present when large joints involved (e.g., knee, ankle); tenderness over sacroiliac joints is common

Mucocutaneous Lesions "Keratoderma blenorrhagica," characterized by hyperkeratotic lesions with erythematous base, usually on extremities (including palms and soles), sometimes in clusters; may resemble psoriasis, both clinically and histologically; pustular component sometimes present; involvement of glans penis in uncircumcised men results in pathognomonic geographic dermatitis ("circinate balanitis"); conjunctivitis; superficial ulcers of oral mucosa

Other Manifestations Fever and malaise occasionally present; uncommon findings (<1 percent of cases) include severe ocular inflammation (iritis, uveitis), heart block or other cardiac arrhythmias, and focal neurologic signs; amyloidosis rarely complicates chronic cases

LABORATORY DIAGNOSIS

No definitive laboratory test; HLA typing recommended by most authorities; evaluate as for NGU and cervicitis, including tests for *C. trachomatis* and *N. gonorrhoeae*; if gastrointestinal symptoms present, evaluate for enteric infection, especially *Shigella, Campylobacter,* and *Yersinia* (Chap. 20); exclude other causes of arthritis (e.g., rheumatoid factor, blood cultures, antinuclear antibody); lumbosacral spine x-rays often show evidence of sacroiliitis; VDRL, HIV serology; if joint effusion present, aspirate synovial fluid and examine for cells, crystals, and culture for bacterial pathogens

DIAGNOSTIC CRITERIA

The American Rheumatism Association defines Reiter's syndrome simply as seronegative arthritis >1 month in duration, associated with urethritis or cervicitis; other causes must be excluded; HLA-B27 haplotype may help confirm diagnosis; if disseminated gonococcal infection or pyogenic infection cannot be excluded, an antibiotic trial may help establish diagnosis

TREATMENT

Treat triggering infection with appropriate antibiotic; no evidence that antibiotic treatment alters course of arthritis or mucocutaneous inflammation; mainstay of arthritis therapy is indomethacin, but newer nonsteroidal anti-inflammatory agents may be helpful; aspirin and glucocorticoids usually not effective; cases should be managed in consultation with an experienced rheumatologist

CONTROL MEASURES

Manage sex partners and report cases as indicated by triggering infection

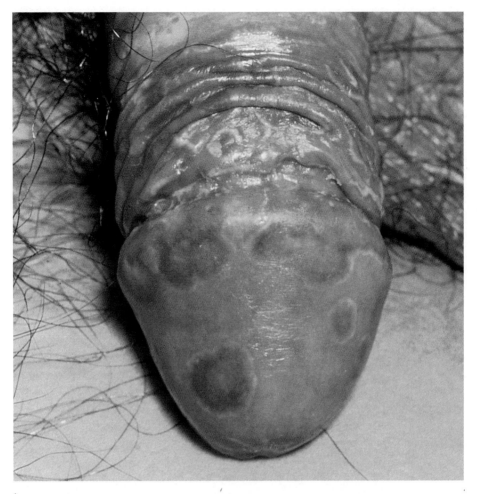

16-1 *Reiter's syndrome: circinate balanitis.* (Reprinted with permission from KK Holmes et al (eds), Sexually Transmitted Diseases, 2d ed. New York, McGraw-Hill, 1990.)

Patient Profile   Age 27, male surgery resident

History   Progressive low back pain and intermittent pain in both heels for 4 weeks; rash involving penis and feet for 3 days; pain and swelling of right knee for 1 day; no genital symptoms, diarrhea, fever, or other symptoms; last sexual exposure 2 months previously

Examination Effusion and decreased range of motion of right knee; tenderness at Achilles tendon insertion points of both heels; hyperkeratotic inflammatory skin lesions of lower extremities; "geographic" rash of penis; no urethral discharge; 50 ml cloudy, straw-colored synovial fluid aspirated from knee

Differential Diagnosis Reiter's syndrome, psoriatic arthritis, ankylosing spondylitis, rheumatoid arthritis, disseminated gonococcal infection

Laboratory Urethral smear showed 10–12 PMNs per 1000 × (oil immersion) field, without gram-negative diplococci; urethral swabs cultured for *C. trachomatis* (positive) and *N. gonorrhoeae* (negative); synovial fluid contained 42,000 leukocytes per mm^3 with 90 percent PMNs, no crystals, negative Gram stain and culture; rheumatoid factor and VDRL negative; spinal and sacroiliac radiographs normal; complete blood count and chemistry panel normal; sedimentation rate 43 mm/h; HLA-B27-positive

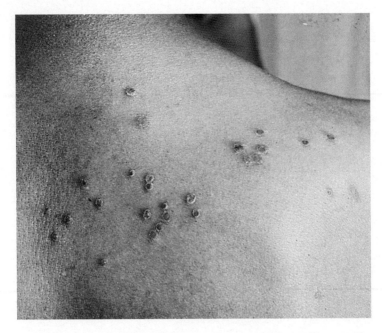

16-2 *Reiter's syndrome: keratoderma blenorrhagica* (Courtesy of Robert Willkens, M.D.)

Diagnosis   Reiter's syndrome

Treatment   Doxycycline 100 mg PO BID for 7 days; indomethacin 150 mg PO TID

Management of Partner   Referred for examination and treatment for chlamydial infection

Comment   Excellent symptomatic response, permitting cessation of indomethacin after 2 months; subsequent chronic but nonlimiting low back pain; repeat sacroiliac x-rays after 1 year showed hypertrophic changes and narrowed joint spaces

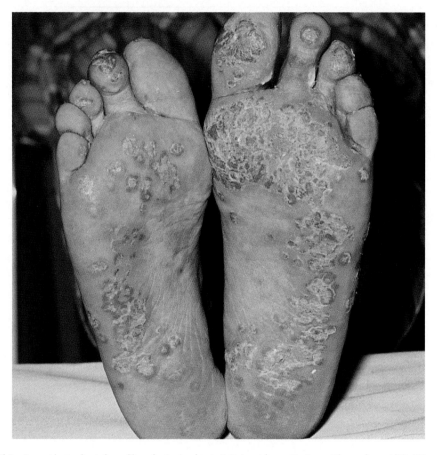

16-3   *Severe plantar keratoderma blenorrhagica in chronic Reiter's syndrome. Compare with secondary syphilis (Fig. 4-14).* (Courtesy of Robert Willkens, M.D.)

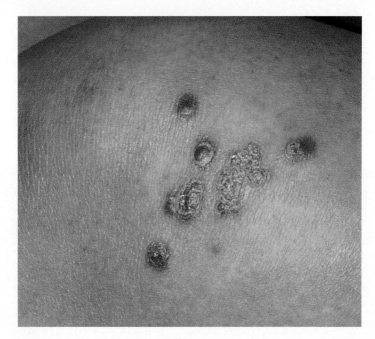

16-4 *Cutaneous lesions consistent with keratoderma blenorrhagica or psoriasis in a woman with acute spondyloarthropathy; the specific diagnosis was never determined.* (Reprinted with permission from KK Holmes et al (eds), Sexually Transmitted Diseases, 2d ed. New York, McGraw-Hill, 1990.)

V CLINICAL STD SYNDROMES

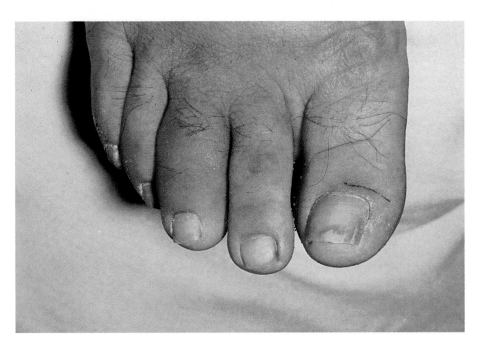

16-5 *Diffuse dactylitis ("sausage toe") of the third digit in a patient with Reiter's syndrome.* (Reprinted with permission from KK Holmes et al (eds), Sexually Transmitted Diseases, 2d ed. New York, McGraw-Hill, 1990.)

ADDITIONAL READING

Handsfield HH, Pollack PS: Arthritis associated with sexually transmitted diseases, in *Sexually Transmitted Diseases,* 2d ed, KK Holmes, et al (eds). New York, McGraw-Hill, 1990, chap 61.

Keat A: Reiter's syndrome and reactive arthritis in perspective. *N Engl J Med* 309:1606, 1983.

Seronegative (reactive) arthropathy: Precipitating factors, editorial. *Lancet* 2:200, 1988.

Chapter 17 Mucopurulent Cervicitis

Mucopurulent cervicitis (MPC) is the female counterpart of urethritis in men. The major cause is *Chlamydia trachomatis*. Gonococcal infection can cause some of the clinical manifestations, but in common usage MPC implies chlamydial or other nongonococcal infection. Some cases are due to herpes simplex virus, usually associated with overt ulcerative cervical or genital lesions. Cervical involvement in trichomoniasis can also produce signs of MPC. As for urethritis in men, the etiology remains obscure for over half the cases. The primary recognized complication is pelvic inflammatory disease. Diagnosis can be difficult, because the clinical and laboratory signs are insensitive and nonspecific. For these reasons, and because the consequences of untreated MPC can be severe, clinicians should maintain a high index of suspicion and a low threshold for treating patients with suspected MPC.

EPIDEMIOLOGY

Incidence and Prevalence Accurate statistics not available; incidence presumably parallels occurrence of chlamydial infection; present in about 20 percent of women in some STD clinics

Transmission As for gonorrhea and chlamydial infection

Age Risk probably highest during adolescence, perhaps due in part to physiologic cervical ectopy (replacement of squamous ectocervical epithelium with columnar endocervical mucosa); ectopy may increase risk by exposing more susceptible endocervical epithelium to infectious agents

Race No known predilection

Other Risk Factors Hormonal contraception and pregnancy are associated with cervical ectopy and may increase risk of MPC

HISTORY

Incubation Period As for chlamydial infection

Symptoms Increased vaginal discharge; intermenstrual bleeding common, especially postcoital spotting; many cases asymptomatic

Epidemiologic History Reflects STD risks; especially common in sexually active adolescents

PHYSICAL EXAMINATION

Various combinations of mucopurulent exudate emanating from cervical os; yellow color of cervical secretions on swab examined outside vagina (positive "swab test"); edema in area of cervical ectopy; apparent rapid appearance of ectopy, due to eversion of inflamed, edematous cervix; endocervical bleeding ("friability") induced by gentle swabbing; cervical tenderness (usually mild) on bimanual examination

LABORATORY DIAGNOSIS

Endocervical Gram-stained smear showing monolayer of ≥20 PMNs per 1000× (oil immersion) microscopic field; PMNs in cervical mucus is valuable sign, because vaginal and ectocervical epithelia lack mucus glands, and mucus denotes endocervical origin; all endocervical specimens must be carefully collected to avoid contamination with vaginal secretions; inflammatory changes on Pap smear are suggestive; obtain tests for *N. gonorrhoeae, C. trachomatis,* trichomoniasis, and yeasts, plus VDRL and test for HSV in selected cases

DIAGNOSTIC CRITERIA

1. Mucopurulent cervical exudate or positive "swab test"
2. Cervical smear with ≥20 PMNs per 1000× microscopic field, or showing PMNs in mucus (not reliable during menses)
3. Edematous cervical ectopy
4. Swab-induced endocervical bleeding
5. History of increased vaginal discharge in absence of clinical and laboratory evidence of vaginal infection

Diagnosis warranted if both mucopurulent cervical exudate and cervical PMNs present (criteria 1 and 2); or by any combination of ≥3 criteria; with fewer criteria, diagnosis possible but not confirmed—test for *C. trachomatis* and *N. gonorrhoeae,* examine sex partners, and reexamine after 1 week

TREATMENT

Doxycycline 100 mg PO BID for 7 days; tetracycline or erythromycin are alternatives, as for NGU and chlamydial infection (Chaps. 3 and 14); if gonorrhea not excluded, precede with ceftriaxone 250 mg IM or other single-dose treatment for gonorrhea (Chap. 2)

CONTROL MEASURES

As for chlamydial infections and gonorrhea; sexual partners should be examined and treated

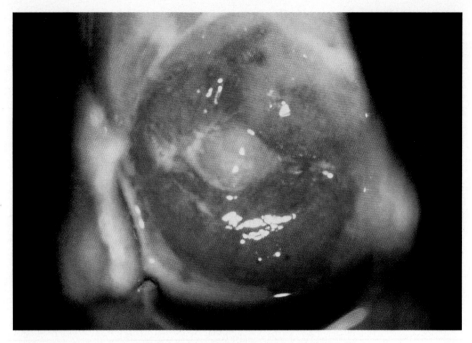

17-1 *Mucopurulent cervicitis: mucopurulent discharge from cervical os.*

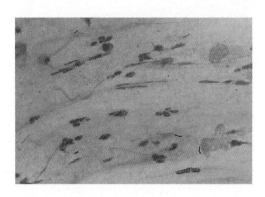

17-2 *Gram-stained smear of cervical secretions in mucopurulent cervicitis, showing PMNs in mucus strands; a few lactobacilli but no gram-negative diplococci are present. Mucus denotes endocervical origin.*

Patient Profile Age 16, high-school student

History Slight increased vaginal discharge for 10 days; responded to partner notification after NGU diagnosed in boyfriend

Examination External genitals normal; cervix showed edematous ectopy, mucopurulent exudate in os, scant bleeding induced by swab

Differential Diagnosis Mucopurulent cervicitis, probably chlamydial; possible gonorrhea, trichomoniasis, herpes

Laboratory Cervical smear showed 20–30 PMNs per oil immersion field, including PMNs in mucus strands; no gram-negative diplococci; vaginal secretions pH 4.0, negative KOH amine odor test; no yeasts, clue cells, or trichomonads seen microscopically; cultures for *C. trachomatis* (positive) and *N. gonorrhoeae* (negative); VDRL, HIV serology (both negative)

Diagnosis Mucopurulent cervicitis due to *C. trachomatis*

Treatment Doxycycline 100 mg PO BID for 7 days

Other Typical case of chlamydial MPC; would have qualified for treatment regardless of history of NGU in partner

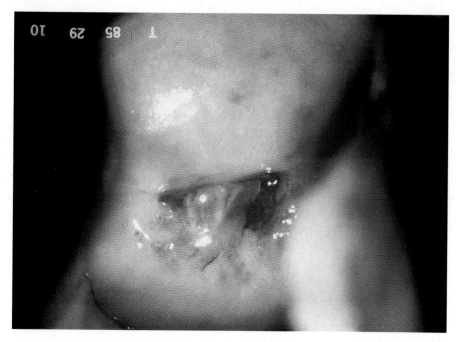

17-3 *Mucopurulent cervicitis due to* Neisseria gonorrhoeae: *Note that mucoid rather than overtly purulent exudate can be seen in gonococcal infection (compare with Figs. 2-6, 3-2, and 17-1).* (Courtesy of Claire E. Stevens.)

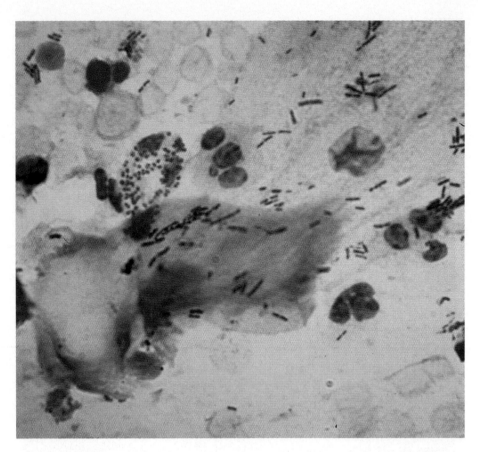

17-4   *Gram-stained smear in gonococcal cervicitis, showing a single PMN with ICGND.* (Courtesy of Claire E. Stevens.)

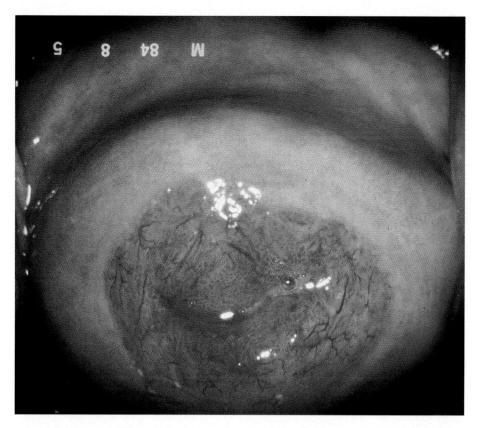

17-5 *Mucopurulent cervicitis due to* Chlamydia trachomatis: *edematous cervical ectopy and scant mucopurlent exudate.* (Courtesy of Claire E. Stevens.)

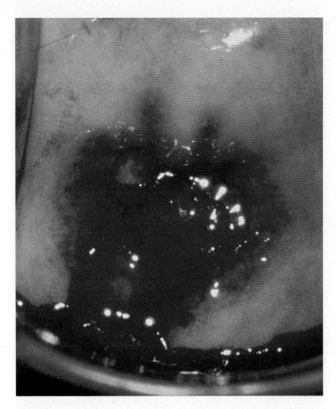

17-6 *Mucopurulent cervicitis; bleeding induced by swab.* (Courtesy of Claire E. Stevens.)

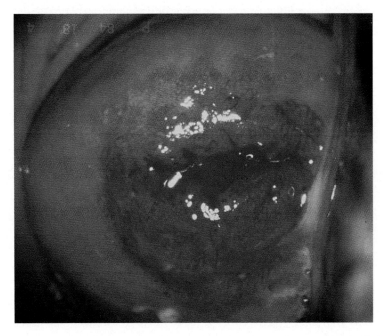

17-7   *Edematous ectopy with incipent endocervical bleeding in a patient with mucopurulent cervicitis; her chief complaint was postcoital bleeding.* (Courtesy of Claire E. Stevens.)

ADDITIONAL READING

Brunham RC et al: Mucopurulent cervicitis: The ignored counterpart in women of urethritis in men. *N Engl J Med* 311:1, 1984.

Holmes KK: Lower genital tract infections in women: Cystitis, urethritis, vulvovaginitis, and cervicitis, in *Sexually Transmitted Diseases,* 2d ed, KK Holmes et al (eds). New York, McGraw-Hill, 1990, chap 46.

Stamm WE: Lower genital tract infections in women. *Infect Dis Clin North Am* 1:179, 1987.

Chapter 18   Vaginal Infections

Vulvovaginal yeast infections, bacterial vaginosis, and trichomoniasis are among the most common reasons for which women seek health care. All sexually active women with trichomoniasis and bacterial vaginosis and some with yeast infections should be routinely evaluated for gonorrhea, chlamydial infection, syphilis, HIV infection, and other STDs.

Yeast infections are usually not sexually acquired; *Candida albicans* and other yeasts commonly colonize the vagina, and a variety of known factors (e.g., suppression of vaginal bacterial flora by antibiotics) and unknown ones result in changes in the growth pattern of these organisms or the immunologic response to them, with resulting inflammation. Vaginal yeast infections are typically associated with vulvitis and with a vigorous PMN response, an important diagnostic feature.

Bacterial vaginosis (BV), formerly called nonspecific vaginitis, is characterized by overgrowth of commensal vaginitis, including *Gardnerella vaginalis, Mobiluncus* sp., *Mycoplasma hominis,* and numerous anaerobic species, and by depletion of facultative vaginal *Lactobacillus* sp. The etiology of these changes is unknown, and it is uncertain whether BV is sexually acquired. No male counterpart has been defined, and treatment of the sex partners has not been shown to influence the rate of recurrence after treatment. Nevertheless, the syndrome is associated with sexual activity and with epidemiologic markers for STD, such as recent intercourse with a new partner and past history of STDs. There is little or no inflammatory response, and leukocytes are not usually found in the vaginal fluid—hence the term vaginosis, not vaginitis. Instead, BV is characterized by "clue cells," vaginal epithelial cells with large numbers of adherent bacteria. BV appears to confer an increased risk of pelvic inflammatory disease, premature labor, and other complications of labor and delivery.

Trichomonas vaginalis is sexually transmitted. The apparent exceptions are usually explained by delayed development of symptoms or by diagnosis of asymptomatic cases several months or years after infection. Symptomatic trichomoniasis is associated with an inflammatory response and with changes in the bacterial flora similar to those of BV. Other STDs, particularly gonorrhea, are especially common in women with recently acquired trichomoniasis.

Other less common causes of vaginal inflammation include retained foreign bodies (e.g., tampons, contraceptive sponges), enterovaginal fistulas, and estrogen deficiency ("atrophic vaginitis"). Physiologic fluctuation in the quantity of vaginal secretions explains many complaints of increased discharge.

EPIDEMIOLOGY

Incidence and Prevalence Reliable community-wide statistics not available; among women attending STD clinics, yeast infections are diagnosed in 20–25 percent, BV in 15–20 percent, and trichomoniasis in 8–12 percent

Transmission Most yeast infections result from chronic colonization; transmission of BV uncertain, but associated with sexual activity; trichomoniasis is sexually acquired, with few if any exceptions

Age Trichomoniasis and BV have age distribution similar to other STDs; trichomoniasis is also seen in older women, reflecting delayed diagnosis of chronic carriage; yeast infections occur at all ages

Sex No known male counterpart to BV; occasional yeast colonization of the penis of partners of women with candidiasis; trichomonas colonizes male urethra or periurethral glands, usually without symptoms, but sometimes causes NGU

Race No special predisposition; trichomoniasis more common in blacks and Hispanics than whites, undoubtedly due to behavioral differences (see Chaps. 2 and 4)

Sexual Orientation Trichomoniasis and BV probably less common in exclusively homosexual women, but accurate data unavailable

Other Risk Factors Antibiotic therapy, diabetes mellitus, and immunodeficiency (e.g., HIV infection) predispose to yeast infection; BV and trichomoniasis correlated with sexual activity

HISTORY

Incubation Period Highly variable for all three syndromes; asymptomatic infections or colonization common

Symptoms
YEAST VULVOVAGINITIS Symptoms due primarily to vulvitis, with external irritation, pruritus, or "external" dysuria due to contact of urine with inflamed labia; discharge usually scant; usually no malodor (contrary to popular belief)
BACTERIAL VAGINOSIS Genital malodor (often described as "fishy") is most common symptom; increased vaginal discharge; many cases asymptomatic
TRICHOMONIASIS Increased discharge and malodor; vulvar pruritus or irritation common, but usually mild

Epidemiologic History For BV and trichomoniasis, history of STD risk factors and markers usually present; for yeast infection, recent use of antibiotics

PHYSICAL EXAMINATION

Yeast Vulvovaginitis Vulvar erythema, sometimes with superficial fissures; scant, clumped, white discharge, adherent to vaginal mucosa is classical, but more homogeneous exudate also is common

Bacterial Vaginosis Scant to moderate discharge, usually white, homogeneous, smoothly coating vaginal walls; usually no erythema or other inflammatory signs

Trichomoniasis Homogeneous discharge, variable in amount, usually purulent in appearance, sometimes foamy; often vaginal mucosal erythema; occasional petechiae on ectocervix ("strawberry cervix"); occasional labial erythema; sometimes tenderness of uterine fundus

LABORATORY DIAGNOSIS

Yeast Infection Vaginal secretions pH ≤ 4.5 (not valid if blood present); no amine odor on alkalinization of secretions with 10% KOH; microscopy (Gram stain or saline mount) demonstrates PMNs and usually both yeasts and pseudomycelia; culture for yeasts usually not helpful, because 25–40 percent of women are colonized

Bacterial Vaginosis Vaginal secretions pH ≥4.7; amine odor with 10% KOH; saline mount or Gram stain shows clue cells, usually without PMNs; Gram stain shows profusion of small, pleomorphic gram-negative and -positive bacilli and cocci and few or no large gram-positive bacilli (*Lactobacillus* sp.)

Trichomoniasis Vaginal secretions pH ≥5.0; motile trichomonads and PMNs; if trichomonads not seen, culture for *T. vaginalis* is useful; clue cells often present; changes in bacterial flora similar to BV

DIAGNOSTIC APPROACH

The first step in evaluating women with vaginal discharge is a careful speculum examination to distinguish whether discharge originates from the cervix (see Chap. 17) or the vagina. The character of the discharge is assessed and the vaginal mucosa and vulva are inspected for inflammatory signs, ulcers, and other lesions. Subsequently, determination of the pH of vaginal secretions, presence or absence of a fishy amine odor on addition of 10% KOH, and microscopic examination (by wet mount, Gram stain, or both) usually permit accurate and rapid office diagnosis. Sometimes culture for *T. vaginalis* is useful. Tests for gonorrhea, chlamydia, and syphilis should be routine, except for reliably monogamous or sexually inactive women with yeast infection.

Table 18-1 summarizes the clinical and laboratory characteristics of these three infections.

TREATMENT

Yeast Vulvovaginitis Any of several vaginal creams or suppositories containing imidazole antifungal antibiotics (e.g., miconazole, clotrimazole, butoconazole, and others), usually administered once daily at bedtime for 3–7 days; single-dose fluconazole 150–200 mg PO is a promising alternative; single-dose topical regimens are unreliable

Bacterial Vaginosis

TREATMENT OF CHOICE   Metronidazole 500 mg PO BID for 7 days

ALTERNATIVES   Clindamycin 300 mg PO BID for 7 days (when metronidazole contraindicated, as in pregnancy); metronidazole 2.0 g PO in a single dose, when compliance with multiple-dose therapy is unlikely (similar short-term efficacy but higher recurrence rate); vaginal administration of 1% clindamycin cream is a promising experimental regimen; tetracyclines, sulfonamides, and other antibiotics have little or no efficacy, either systemically or topically; douching is ineffective and potentially harmful (see Chap. 19); commercially available *Lactobacillus* preparations have not been shown to be effective

Trichomoniasis   Metronidazole 2.0 g PO (single dose); metronidazole 500 mg PO BID for 7 days (if single-dose treatment fails)

Management of Sex Partners

YEAST INFECTION   Usually not indicated, unless history suggests penile dermatitis

BACTERIAL VAGINOSIS   Evaluate for STD; routine treatment not indicated; however, some clinicians empirically treat partners (usually with amoxicillin or metronidazole) of patients with frequently recurring BV

TRICHOMONIASIS   Evaluate for STD; metronidazole 2.0 g PO in a single dose; treatment usually should not be given to partners who are not examined

Table 18-1
Diagnostic Features of Vaginal Infection in Premenopausal Adults

	NORMAL	YEAST VULVOVAGINITIS	TRICHOMONAL VAGINITIS	BACTERIAL VAGINOSIS
Typical symptoms	None	Vulvar itching and/or irritation, increased discharge	Profuse purulent discharge; sometimes vulvar itching	Malodor, slightly increased discharge
Discharge:				
Amount	Variable; usually scant	Scant to moderate	Profuse	Scant to moderate
Color*	Clear or white	White or yellow	Yellow	Usually white
Consistency	Nonhomogeneous, floccular	Clumped; adherent plaques	Homogeneous; sometimes foamy	Homogeneous, low viscosity; smoothly coats vaginal mucosa
Inflammation of vulvar or vaginal epithelium	None	Erythema of vaginal epithelium, introitus; vulvar dermatitis common	Erythema of vaginal and vulvar epithelium; sometimes petechiae of ectocervix	None
pH of vaginal fluid†	Usually ≤4.5	Usually ≤4.5	Usually ≥5.0	Usually ≥4.7
Amine (fishy) odor with 10% KOH	None	None	Present	Present
Microscopy‡	Normal epithelial cells; lactobacilli predominate	Leukocytes, epithelial cells; yeasts or pseudomycelia (up to 80%)	Leukocytes; motile trichomonads seen in 80–90% of symptomatic patients, less often in absence of symptoms	Clue cells; few leukocytes; profuse mixed flora with few or no lactobacilli

* Color of discharge is best determined by examining vaginal discharge against a white background.

† pH determination is not useful if blood is present.

‡ To detect fungal elements, vaginal fluid is digested with 10% KOH prior to microscopic examination; to examine for other features, fluid is mixed (1:1) with physiologic saline. Gram stain also is excellent for detecting yeasts and pseudomycelia and for distinguishing normal flora from the mixed flora seen in bacterial vaginosis, but is insensitive for detection of *T. vaginalis*.

SOURCE: Modified from KK Holmes et al (eds), *Sexually Transmitted Diseases*, 2d ed, New York, McGraw-Hill, 1990.

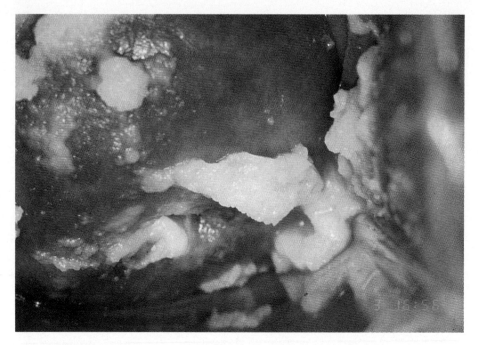

18-1   *Clumped vaginal exudate in vulvovaginitis due to* Candida albicans. (Courtesy of Claire E. Stevens.)

Patient Profile   Age 20, college student, sexually active with a single partner

History   Vulvar itching and increased vaginal discharge for 2 days; treated 10 days earlier with an unknown antibiotic for bacterial urinary tract infection

Examination   Vulvar erythema; white discharge in patches on cervix and vaginal mucosa; otherwise normal

Differential Diagnosis   Yeast infection; trichomoniasis, BV, and MPC unlikely

Laboratory   Vaginal pH 4.0; amine odor test negative; Gram stain and saline mount showed PMNs, yeasts, and pseudomycelia; screening test for *C. trachomatis* (negative)

Diagnosis   Yeast vulvovaginitis, probably due to *Candida albicans*

Treatment   Clotrimazole 100 mg vaginal cream daily at bedtime for 7 days

Management of Sex Partner   Patient advised to ascertain that her partner has no penile rash or other genital symptoms

Other   Screening tests for other STDs optional in view of recent antibiotic therapy and reliable history of monogamous sexual relationship

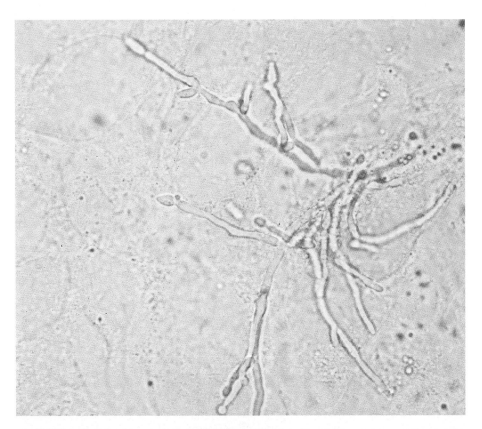

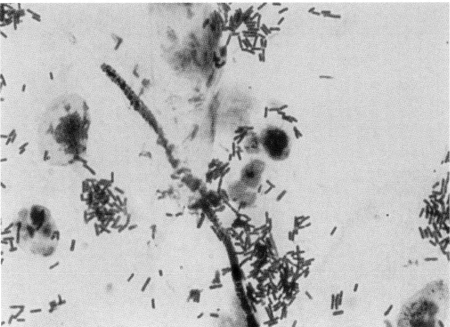

18-2　*Yeast vulvovaginitis. a. Potassium hydroxide digest of vaginal secretions, showing pseudohyphae of* Candida albicans. (Courtesy of David A. Eschenbach, M.D.) *b. Gram-stained smear of vaginal secretions, showing a mottled, gram-positive pseudohypha of* Candida albicans *and multiple* Lactobacillus *morphotypes.* (Courtesy of Sharon L. Hillier, Ph.D.)

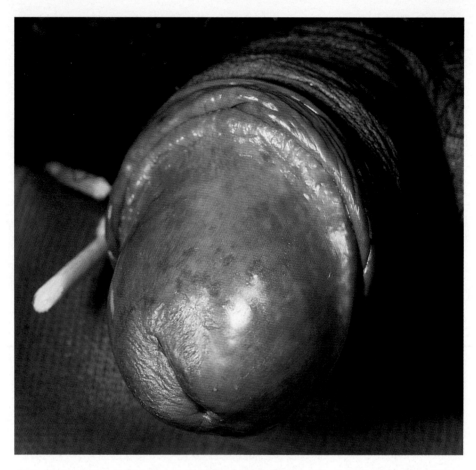

18-3   *Punctuate lesions of glans penis due to* Candida *balanitis in the partner of a woman with yeast vulvovaginitis.*

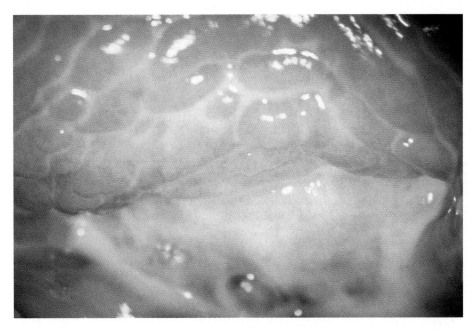

18-4 *Bacterial vaginosis: white, homogeneous discharge smoothly coating the vaginal mucosa. Also see Fig. 9-2.* (Courtesy of Claire E. Stevens.)

Patient Profile Age 22, single, photographer's assistant

History Increased vaginal discharge with a "strong" odor for 1 week; began a new sexual relationship one month previously

Examination Homogeneous white vaginal secretions at introitus and coating vaginal walls; cervix showed small area of ectopy, with cloudy mucus in os; bimanual examination normal

Differential Diagnosis BV, trichomoniasis, yeast infection, MPC, gonorrhea, physiologic discharge

Laboratory Vaginal secretions pH 5.0; amine odor with addition of 10% KOH; saline preparation showed clue cells, no trichomonads, rare leukocytes; Gram stain of cervical secretions showed 2–4 PMNs per 1000× field, without ICGND; cervical cultures for *C. trachomatis* and *N. gonorrhoeae*, VDRL (all negative); declined HIV testing

Diagnosis Bacterial vaginosis

Treatment Metronidazole 500 mg PO BID for 7 days

Management of Sex Partner(s) Advised to refer her partner for STD evaluation; partner does not require treatment if examination normal and STD tests negative

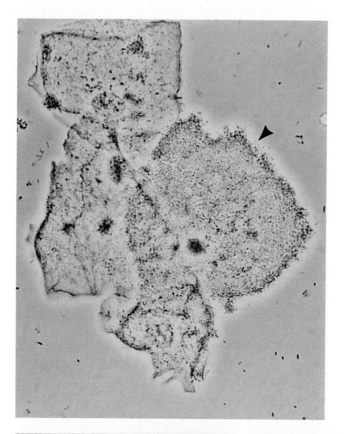

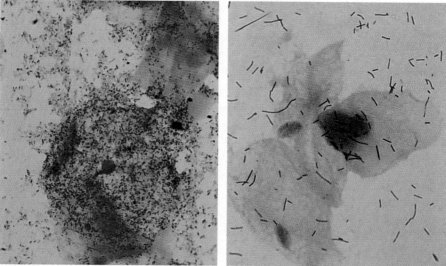

18-5   *Bacterial vaginosis. a. Clue cells (arrow) adjacent to vaginal epithelial cells; clue cells have indistinct, ragged margins and a refractile, granular appearance due to large numbers of adherent bacteria.* (Courtesy of David A. Eschenbach, M.D.) *b. Gram-stained smears of secretions in bacterial vaginosis (left) and normal vaginal secretions (right); the bacterial vaginosis smear shows a clue cell, numerous pleomorphic bacteria consistent with* Gardnerella vaginalis *and anaerobes, and absence of large, gram-positive bacilli* (Lactobacillus *sp.*); *the normal smear contains epithelial cells without adherent bacteria and predominant* Lactobacillus *sp.* (Courtesy of Sharon L. Hillier, Ph.D.)

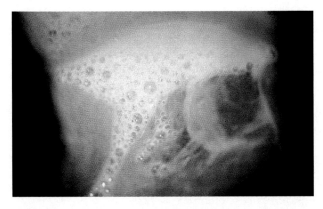

18-6 *Purulent vaginal discharge in trichomonal vaginitis; bubbles due to gas production by anaerobic bacteria, although typical, are seen in a minority of cases.* (Courtesy of Claire E. Stevens.)

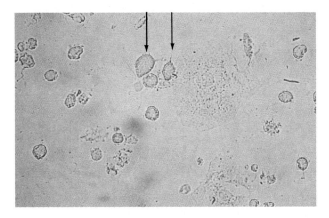

18-7 *Saline wet mount of vaginal secretions in trichomonal vaginitis, showing two* T. vaginalis *(arrows), leukocytes, and a normal vaginal epithelial cell; in actual use, trichomonads are distinguished from leukocytes primarily by their characteristic motility.*

Patient Profile   Age 24, single, unemployed, referred from drug rehabilitation facility

History   Increased vaginal discharge and slight vulvar itching for 2 weeks; one partner for 6 months

Examination   External genitals normal; vaginal mucosa slightly erythematous; profuse yellow discharge; cervix normal; slight tenderness of uterine fundus; no adnexal tenderness or masses

Differential Diagnosis   Trichomoniasis, gonorrhea, chlamydial infection, BV, yeast infection

Laboratory   Vaginal pH 5.5; amine odor test positive; saline preparaton showed leukocytes, motile trichomonads, clue cells; endocervical Gram stain showed 20 PMNs per 1000 × field, without gram-negative diplococci; cultures for *C. trachomatis* (negative) and *N. gonorrhoeae* (positive); VDRL, HIV antibody test (both negative)

Diagnosis   Trichomonal vaginitis; gonorrhea

Treatment   Metronidazole 2.0 g PO, single dose; called back after *N. gonorrhoeae* isolated and given ceftriaxone 250 mg IM (doxycycline optional, because chlamydia culture negative)

Management of Partner   Contacted; treated for trichomoniasis and gonorrhea

Comment   Trichomoniasis commonly associated with other STDs; endocervical PMNs could be due to trichomoniasis, gonorrhea, or both

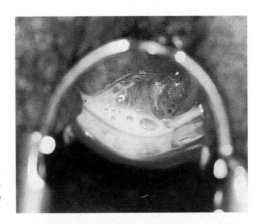

18-8 *Vaginal discharge (with bubbles) due to tricho-moniasis; cervical discharge and edematous ectopy due to mucopurulent cervicitis also are present.*

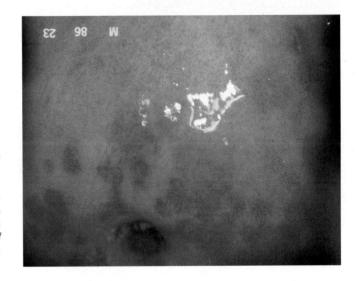

18-9 *Cervical petechiae ("strawberry cervix"), an uncommon but classical manifestation of trichomoniasis.* (Reprinted with permission from KK Holmes et al (eds), *Sexually Transmitted Diseases,* 2d ed. New York, McGraw-Hill, 1990.)

ADDITIONAL READING

Eschenbach DA et al: Diagnosis and clinical manifestations of bacterial vaginosis. *Am J Obstet Gynecol* 158:19, 1988.

Hillier S, Holmes KK: Bacterial vaginosis, in *Sexually Transmitted Diseases,* 2d ed, KK Holmes et al (eds). New York, McGraw-Hill, 1990, chap 47.

Holmes KK: Lower genital tract infections in women: Cystitis, urethritis, vulvovaginitis, and cervicitis, in *Sexually Transmitted Diseases,* 2d ed, KK Holmes et al (eds). New York, McGraw-Hill, 1990, chap 46.

Lossick JG: Treatment of sexually transmitted vaginosis/vaginitis. *Rev Infect Dis* 12(suppl 6):S665, 1990.

Rein MF, Müller M: *Trichomonas vaginalis* infection and trichomoniasis, in *Sexually Transmitted Diseases,* 2d ed, KK Holmes et al (eds). New York, McGraw-Hill, 1990, chap 43.

Sobel JD: Vulvovaginal candidiasis, in *Sexually Transmitted Diseases,* 2d ed, KK Holmes et al (eds). New York, McGraw-Hill, 1990, chap 45.

Wølner-Hanssen P et al: Clinical manifestations of vaginal trichomoniasis. *JAMA* 261:571, 1989.

Chapter 19 Pelvic Inflammatory Disease

Pelvic inflammatory disease (PID) is the most common serious complication of STD. PID is defined as salpingitis, often accompanied by endometritis or secondary pelvic peritonitis, that results from ascending genital infection, unrelated to childbirth or surgical manipulation. The primary threat of PID is tubal scarring that leads to infertility and ectopic pregnancy. PID is often clinically severe, with tubovarian abscess, overt peritonitis, prominent fever, and other systemic symptoms. However, most cases are relatively mild. Asymptomatic salpingitis appears to be common and can result in tubal scarring and obstruction, as evidenced by the frequent absence of a past history of PID or abdominal pain in chlamydia-seropositive women with tubal-factor infertility or ectopic pregnancy. Recent data suggest that vaginal douching is a potent independent risk factor for PID. Douching has not been shown to treat any infection effectively and therefore should not be prescribed, and sexually active women should be discouraged from hygienic or prophylactic douching.

Over the past decade the proportion of PID cases caused by *N. gonorrhoeae* compared with *C. trachomatis* has declined in most industrialized countries, reflecting the relative incidences of these infections. Numerous other bacteria contribute to PID, including *Mycoplasma hominis* and various aerobic and anaerobic components of the vaginal flora. It is probable that any of several inflammatory events involving the endocervix (e.g., gonorrhea, chlamydial infection, or other causes of mucopurulent cervicitis) may result in ascending infection with the primary pathogen, vaginal bacteria, or both. Bacterial vaginosis is often present and may predispose to PID by virtue of the 100- to 1000-fold increased concentration of aerobic and anaerobic bacteria associated with this syndrome. The specific bacterial pathogens are not usually known, and treatment of all patients should be adequate for gonorrhea, chlamydial infection, and a mixed aerobic and anaerobic flora.

EPIDEMIOLOGY

Incidence and Prevalence   An estimated 600,000 to 1 million cases occur annually in the United States; diagnosed in 2–5 percent of women in STD clinics; PID is the most common cause of female infertility and ectopic pregnancy

Transmission   As for *N. gonorrhoeae, C. trachomatis,* and MPC

Age   Markedly increased risk in sexually active adolescents compared with women >20 years old, probably due to both behavioral and physiologic factors

Race   As for gonorrhea and chlamydial infection

Sexual Orientation   Rare in exclusively homosexual women

Other Risk Factors   Socioeconomic and behavioral markers of STD risk; intrauterine device (IUD) for contraception; previous PID; hormonal contraception apparently reduces risk, especially of chlamydial PID; vaginal douching increases risk

HISTORY

Incubation Period   Varies from 1–2 days to several weeks or months

Symptoms   Low abdominal pain nearly universal in symptomatic cases; most cases have symptoms of lower genital tract infection (vaginal discharge, malodor, dysuria, etc.); dyspareunia; menorrhagia; intermenstrual bleeding; occasional right upper quadrant abdominal pain; fever, chills, malaise, nausea and vomiting suggest severe infection; many cases clinically mild or asymptomatic

Epidemiologic History   Young age (15–25 years) is typical; most patients have recent new sex partner or other STD risks

PHYSICAL EXAMINATION

Pelvic adnexal tenderness, usually bilateral; uterine fundal and cervical-motion tenderness; palpable adnexal mass(es) often present, especially in severe cases; lower quadrant abdominal tenderness, sometimes with rebound tenderness or other peritoneal signs; right upper quadrant tenderness sometimes present, due to perihepatitis (Fitz-Hugh–Curtis syndrome); evidence of MPC or BV usually present; fever in severe cases

LABORATORY DIAGNOSIS

Lower Genital Tract Infection   Most patients have laboratory manifestations of MPC, BV, or both (see Chaps. 17 and 18)

Microbiology   Endocervical cultures for *N. gonorrhoeae* and *C. trachomatis;* if laparoscopy done, culture tubal aspirate or peritoneal exudate for *N. gonorrhoeae, C. trachomatis,* and aerobic and anaerobic bacteria

Other Tests   Leukocyte count, sedimentation rate, or C-reactive protein may be elevated or normal; these are indicators of clinical severity, but normal results do not rule out PID; perform VDRL and recommend HIV testing for all patients; pelvic ultrasound examination sometimes helpful; laparoscopy indicated in severe cases, if diagnosis uncertain, or if inadequate response to initial antibiotic therapy; endometrial biopsy can be helpful by documenting endometritis, which is usually present in PID

DIAGNOSTIC CRITERIA

Combined clinical, epidemiologic, and laboratory findings; only two-thirds of patients with clinically diagnosed PID have laparoscopic evidence of it; however, some of these cases may reflect early or mild salpingitis without visible serosal erythema or tubal edema

TREATMENT

Principles   Treat all suspected cases while awaiting diagnostic confirmation; routinely cover *N. gonorrhoeae, C. trachomatis, M. hominis,* and mixed aerobic and anaerobic bacteria, regardless of pathogens identified in patient or sex partner; even clinically mild cases should be promptly treated; some authorities recommend inpatient treatment with IV antibiotics, even for mild cases, but hospitalization often precluded by social and financial constraints

Recommended Regimens

INPATIENT TREATMENT   Two regimens are recommended: Use regimen A when chlamydial or gonococcal infection is likely; regimen B is preferred by some experts when predominant aerobic/anaerobic infection is most likely (e.g., IUD-related PID in a woman at low risk for STD)

- *Regimen A:* Doxycycline 100 mg IV every 12 h, plus either cefotetan 2.0 g IV every 12 h or cefoxitin 2.0 g IV every 6 h; continue until at least 48 h after onset of clinical improvement, then give doxycycline 100 mg PO BID to complete 14 days total therapy
- *Regimen B:* Clindamycin 900 mg IV every 8 h, plus either gentamicin or to-bramycin, 2.0 mg/kg body weight as loading dose, then 1.5 mg/kg every 8 h; continue both until at least 48 h after onset of clinical improvement, then give doxycycline 100 mg PO BID, or clindamycin 450 mg PO QID, or both, to complete 14 days total therapy

OUTPATIENT TREATMENT

- Ceftriaxone 250 mg IM or cefoxitin 2.0 g IM plus probenecid 1.0 g PO; plus doxycycline 100 mg PO BID for 14 days; for severe cases with high probability of resistant anaerobic infection, add metronidazole 1.0 g PO BID or clindamycin 450 mg PO QID (e.g., when hospitalization recommended but impractical)

Supportive Therapy Promptly remove IUD, if present; bedrest may speed subjective improvement in severe cases; analgesics as needed; sexual abstention for at least 2 weeks

Follow-up Reexamine outpatients at 1- to 3-day intervals until improved; clinical progression at any time or failure to improve within 3–4 days is indication for hospitalization for laparoscopy and parenteral therapy; after improvement begins, continue to follow weekly until resolved

CONTROL MEASURES

Management of Sex Partners Examine all partners, even if apparently at low risk for STD (e.g., IUD-related PID in an apparently monogamous patient); unless sexual acquisition can be excluded with certainty, treat partner for presumptive gonorrhea and chlamydial infection

Reporting Some states require reporting of all PID, regardless of etiology

Counseling Counsel patient about sexually transmitted nature of PID, risks for infertility (15–30 percent for each episode of PID, depending on severity) and ectopic pregnancy, and importance of avoiding future episodes; avoid nonspecific terms such as "infected ovarian cyst" and others that minimize the sexually transmitted nature of PID

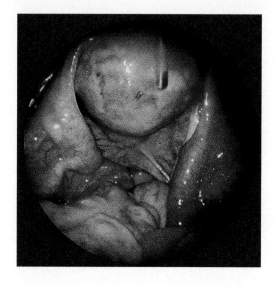

19-1 *Laparoscopic view of pelvic structures in mild acute PID (not from patient described); uterus (under probe) is normal; left fallopian tube (left side of figure) has minimal edema with reddened, agglutinated fimbria; right tube is mildly swollen and erythematous; yellow-green purulent exudate is seen in cul-de-sac.* (Courtesy of David E. Soper, M.D.)

Patient Profile   Age 18, grocery clerk

History   Increased vaginal discharge for 10 days; mild low abdominal pain and dyspareunia for 4 days, severe pain for 1 day; no fever or chills; monogamous with current boyfriend for 3 months

Examination   Afebrile; bilateral lower quadrant abdominal tenderness, without rebound; edematous cervical ectopy and mucopurulent cervical exudate; homogeneous gray vaginal fluid; moderate tenderness of cervix, uterine fundus, and adnexal regions bilaterally; left adnexal "fullness," without overt mass

Differential Diagnosis   PID, ectopic pregnancy, endometriosis, appendicitis, urinary tract infection, colitis

Laboratory   Findings consistent with BV and MPC; WBC 8600 per mm^3 with normal differential; ESR 35 mm/h; endocervical culture positive for *C. trachomatis,* negative for *N. gonorrhoeae;* VDRL and HIV serology negative

Diagnosis   Pelvic inflammatory disease

Treatment   Ceftriaxone 250 mg IM plus doxycycline 100 mg PO BID for 14 days

Management of Sex Partner   Advised to refer partner for examination and treatment; partner found to have asymptomatic chlamydial NGU

Other   Reexamined 2 days later, pain improved, with reduced adnexal tenderness; counseled regarding STD prevention and risks of infertility and ectopic pregnancy

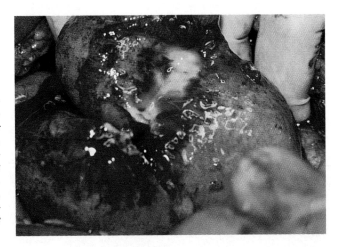

19-2 *Tuboovarian abscess in severe PID (not from patient described); bilobed structure in lower half of figure is pyosalpinx/abscess, which has been dissected from uterine fundus; purulent exudate is present between abscess and uterus.* (Courtesy of David E. Soper, M.D.; reprinted with permission from DE Soper, *Am J Obstet Gynecol* 164:1370, 1991.)

Patient Profile   Age 32, married schoolteacher

History   Intermittent mild low abdominal pain and vaginal discharge since IUD inserted 4 months earlier; severe abdominal pain, fever, chills, nausea, and vomiting for 1 day; monogamous

Examination   Temperature 39.2°C orally; bilateral lower quadrant direct and rebound abdominal tenderness; IUD string and profuse mucopurulent cervical discharge; severe generalized pelvic tenderness, with suggestion of right adnexal mass (inadequate examination due to tenderness and guarding)

Differential Diagnosis   PID, appendicitis, ectopic pregnancy, severe endometriosis

Laboratory   Stat pelvic ultrasound showed 6 × 8-cm fluid-filled mass with internal echoes and small effusion in cul-de-sac; WBC 14,700 per mm^3 with 80 percent PMNs; ESR 50 mm/h; cervical Gram stain and vaginal saline mount showed large numbers of PMNs, moderate clue cells, no trichomonads or yeasts; vaginal pH 5.0, KOH amine odor positive; negative cultures for *N. gonorrhoeae* and *C. trachomatis;* two blood cultures sent (later reported negative); VDRL negative

Diagnosis   PID with tuboovarian abscess, associated with IUD

Treatment   Patient hospitalized; IUD removed; treated with IV clindamycin and gentamicin

Clinical Course   Slow clinical improvement; abscess apparently unchanged on ultrasound 4 days later, drained through cul-de-sac under local anesthesia, with rapid improvement thereafter; discharged on day 7 on clindamycin 450 mg PO QID for 10 more days

Management of Sex Partner   Husband referred for examination; gave reliable history of monogamy; urethral examination normal; negative cultures for *C. trachomatis* and *N. gonorrhoeae;* not treated

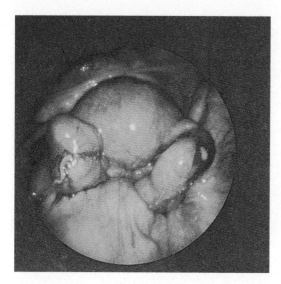

19-3 *Bilateral pyosalpinx in severe PID; pus is seen exuding from left tube after needle aspiration for culture.* (Courtesy of David E. Soper, M.D.; reprinted with permission from DE Soper, *Am J Obstet Gynecol* 164:1370, 1991.)

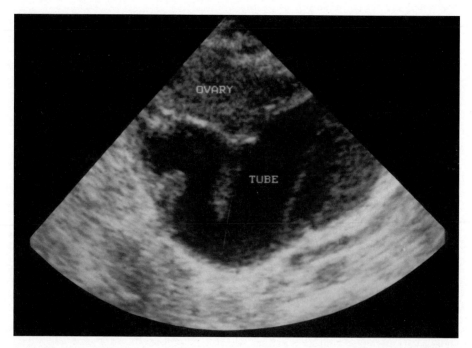

19-4 *Pelvic ultrasound examination in acute PID with pyosalpinx.* (Courtesy of Faye Laing, M.D.)

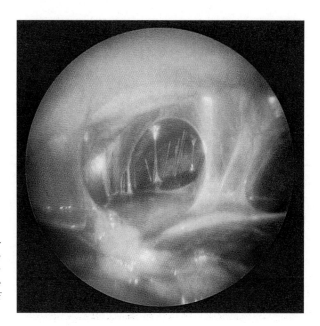

19-5 *Adhesions between liver capsule and parietal peritoneum in a woman with acute perihepatitis (Fitz-Hugh-Curtis syndrome) due to* C. trachomatis. *(Courtesy of David E. Soper, M.D.)*

ADDITIONAL READING

Peterson HB et al: Pelvic inflammatory disease: Review of treatment options. *Rev Infect Dis* 12(suppl 6):S656, 1990.

Soper DE: Diagnosis and laparoscopic grading of acute salpingitis. *Am J Obstet Gynecol* 164:1370, 1991.

Sweet RL: Pelvic inflammatory disease and infertility in women. *Infect Dis Clin North Am* 1:199, 1987.

Weström L, Mårdh P-A: Acute pelvic inflammatory disease, in *Sexually Transmitted Diseases,* 2d ed, KK Holmes et al (eds). New York, McGraw-Hill, 1990, chap 49.

Wølner-Hanssen P et al: Association between vaginal douching and acute pelvic inflammatory disease. *JAMA* 263:1936, 1990.

Chapter 20 Proctitis and Enteric Infections

Several gastrointestinal infections are sexually transmissible. Sexually acquired proctitis occurs by direct inoculation through anal intercourse or perineal contamination with cervicovaginal secretions and is usually due to *N. gonorrhoeae, C. trachomatis,* herpes simplex virus, or occasionally *T. pallidum*. Enteritis, or small intestinal infection, can be acquired through sexual practices that foster fecal-oral contamination. The most commonly recognized sexually transmitted enteritis is giardiasis, but undoubtedly viral enteric pathogens can also be transmitted sexually. Sexually acquired acute colitis or proctocolitis can result from either fecal-oral contamination (e.g., amebiasis, shigellosis) or rectal inoculation (e.g., lymphogranuloma venereum). *Campylobacter* infection and salmonellosis, acquired by the fecal-oral route, typically result in manifestations of enteritis, colitis, or both (enterocolitis). Although all sexually active persons are at risk for these infections, they have been most commonly recognized among homosexually active men. There is little clinical distinction between these and nonsexually acquired intestinal disorders such as inflammatory bowel disease, ischemic colitis, and food- or waterborne gastrointestinal infections.

EPIDEMIOLOGY

Incidence of Prevalence   Reliable statistics not available

Transmission   Fecal-oral or rectal inoculation

Age, Sex, Race   Reflective of sexual activity patterns

Sexual Orientation   Most common in homosexually active men with multiple partners

Other Risk Factors   Influenced by specific sexual practices (e.g., anal intercourse, oral-anal contact)

HISTORY

Incubation Period   Variable, depending on specific infection

Symptoms

- *Enteritis:* Predominantly diarrhea, usually without cramps; sometimes nausea, vomiting, anorexia, flatulence, weight loss, fever
- *Proctitis:* Various combinations of anorectal discharge, pain, tenesmus, constipation, bleeding; anal or perianal lesions (herpes, syphilis); fever and other systemic symptoms uncommon, except for primary herpes and LGV
- *Colitis:* Diarrhea, sometimes bloody, usually accompanied by abdominal cramps; fever and other systemic symptoms common
- *Protocolitis, enterocolitis:* Symptoms of both components of the syndrome

Epidemiologic History   History of exposure or high-risk sexual practices

PHYSICAL EXAMINATION

Enteritis Nonspecific; abdominal tenderness, enhanced bowel sounds, or evidence of weight loss sometimes present

Proctitis Anal or perianal lesions consistent with herpes or syphilis; various combinations of rectal mucosal erythema, purulent exudate, edema, and ulcerative or petechial lesions observed by anoscopy or proctosigmoidoscopy; bleeding may be induced by swabbing rectal mucosa ("wipe test")

Colitis Abdominal tenderness, usually maximal in left lower quadrant; fever commonly present; anoscopy may show evidence of proctitis; sigmoidoscopy or colonoscopy may be indicated to evaluate extent of involvement

LABORATORY DIAGNOSIS

Enteritis Stool culture and examination for ova and parasites; "string test" to obtain duodenal secretions for microscopic examination for *Giardia lamblia* is useful when stool examination is negative

Proctitis Routinely sample anal canal or rectal mucosa (preferably with anoscopic visualization) for Gram-stained smear and culture or antigen-detection tests for *N. gonorrhoeae, C. trachomatis,* and HSV; VDRL and HIV serology; dark-field examination if ulcerative lesions present; rectal mucosal biopsy sometimes required for diagnosis

Colitis As for proctitis; examine stool for leukocytes; stool culture and test for ova and parasites; rectal or colonic biopsy sometimes indicated

TREATMENT

Enteritis
GIARDIASIS Quinacrine 100 mg PO TID for 7 days; or metronidazole 500 mg PO TID for 7 days
SALMONELLOSIS Most cases not treated with antibiotics
CAMPYLOBACTER ENTERITIS/ENTEROCOLITIS Erythromycin 250 mg PO QID for 5–7 days; or ciprofloxacin 500 mg PO BID for 5–7 days (ciprofloxacin also treats shigellosis)

Proctitis Treat according to specific etiology (see Chaps. 2–4, 7); for patients without herpes or syphilis, treat with ceftriaxone plus doxycycline, as for uncomplicated gonorrhea, pending microbiologic test results

Colitis
AMEBIASIS Most cases in homosexual men are due to nonpathogenic strains and do not require treatment; treat prominent colitis with metronidazole 750 mg PO TID for 5–10 days, plus iodoquinol (diiodohydroxyquin) 650 mg PO TID or 3 weeks
SHIGELLOSIS Depends on susceptibility of isolate; in most settings sulfamethoxazole/trimethoprim 800/160 mg ("double strength" tablet) PO BID or ciprofloxacin 500 mg PO BID for 3–5 days are reasonable empiric therapies pending susceptibility tests; ciprofloxacin also treats *Campylobacter*
LGV PROCTOCOLITIS Doxycycline 100 mg PO BID for 2–3 weeks; see Chap. 3

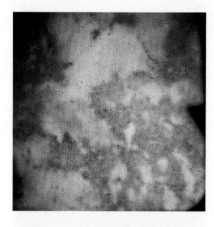

20-1 *Rectal mucosal ulcerations and exudate due to amebic proctocolitis, viewed by fiberoptic sigmoidoscopy; herpetic proctitis produces a similar appearance.* (Courtesy of Thomas Quinn, M.D.)

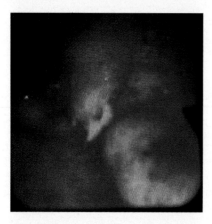

20-2 *Gonococcal proctitis, with purulent exudate and swab-induced mucosal bleeding (positive "wipe test"), viewed by fiberoptic sigmoidoscopy.* (Courtesy of Thomas Quinn, M.D.)

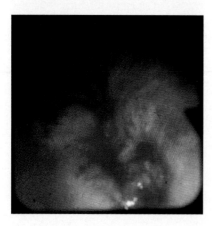

20-3 *Mucosal edema and petechiae in chlamydial proctitis, viewed by fiberoptic sigmoidoscopy.* (Courtesy of Thomas Quinn, M.D.)

V CLINICAL STD SYNDROMES

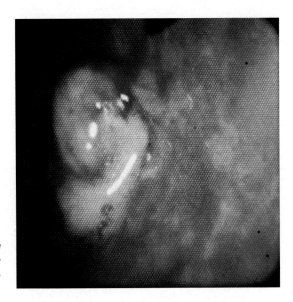

20-4 *Inflammatory pseudopolyp of the rectum in amebic proctocolitis, viewed by fiberoptic sigmoidoscopy.* (Courtesy of Thomas Quinn, M.D.)

ADDITIONAL READING

Quinn TC, Stamm WE: Proctitis, proctocolitis, enteritis, and esophagitis in homosexual men, in *Sexually Transmitted Diseases,* 2d ed, KK Holmes et al (eds). New York, McGraw-Hill, 1990, chap 55.

Rompalo AM, Quinn TC: Sexually transmitted enteric and rectal infections in homosexual men. *Infect Dis Clin North Am* 1:235, 1987.

Chapter 21 Nonsexually Transmitted Genital Dermatoses

Numerous nonsexually transmitted dermatologic disorders commonly involve the genitals. In addition, sexually active persons with genital lesions often present with suspicion or fear of an STD. Although it is beyond the scope of this book to provide a comprehensive review, some examples are presented.

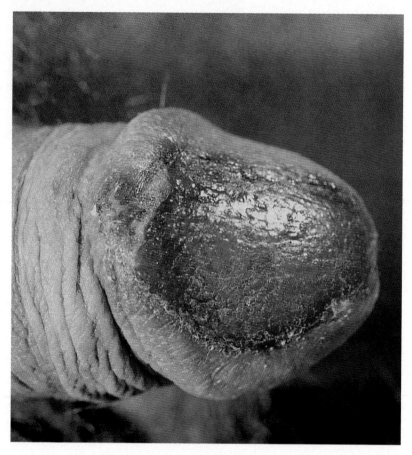

21-1 *Fixed drug eruption of penis.*

Patient Profile Age 25, unmarried male laborer

History Treated 9 days earlier with tetracycline for nongonococcal urethritis; burning pain and "weeping sore" of penis for 3 days beginning on final day of tetracycline therapy

Examination   Superficial sloughing of epidermis of glans penis

Diagnosis   Fixed drug eruption due to tetracycline

Treatment   Local hygiene

Comment   Fixed drug eruptions are localized allergic reactions to systemic therapy and commonly affect the genitals; tetracyclines are among the most common causes, so genital fixed drug eruptions are relatively common among patients with STD or at risk; typically begin after 7–10 days of exposure to allergen, often after treatment is complete; clinical findings and natural course are similar to those of second degree burn, with superficial pain and erythema followed by bulla formation and sloughing; healing occurs without scarring; aside from cessation of offending drug, treatment is supportive; some authorities prescribe topical steroids for lesions diagnosed before bulla formation; other common causes include metronidazole, sulfonamides, and nonsteroidal anti-inflammatory agents, but virtually all drug classes have been implicated

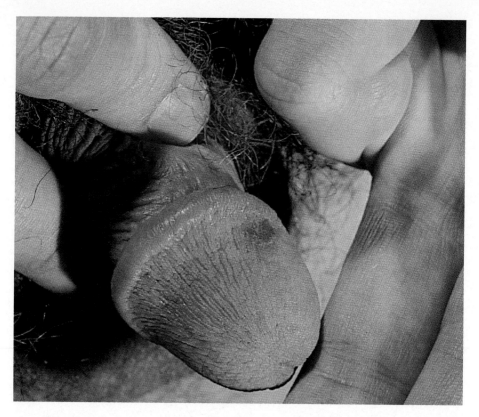

21-2 *Fixed drug eruption: sharply demarcated erythematous lesions of glans penis and finger web in a patient treated with doxycycline for NGU.*

V   CLINICAL STD SYNDROMES

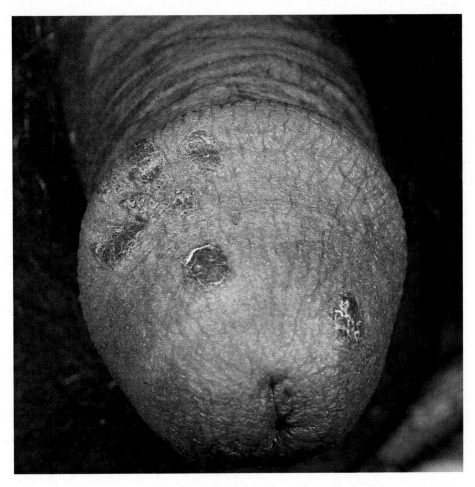

21-3 *Psoriasis of penis.*

Patient Profile Age 24, male graduate student

History Painless penile lesion for 5 days, beginning 2 weeks after intercourse with a new partner; no other rash or skin lesions; no recent drug therapy

Examination Irregular erythematous papulosquamous lesion of glans penis; no lymphadenopathy

Differential Diagnosis   Nonsexually transmitted dermatosis (psoriasis, impetigo, candidiasis, contact dermatitis, etc.); syphilis, herpes, chancroid less likely

Laboratory   VDRL negative; *C. trachomatis* culture negative

Other Information   Patient's sex partner examined, no STD; 2 weeks after presentation, a 1.5-cm hyperkeratotic, exfoliating, erythematous plaque became apparent on scalp

Diagnosis   Psoriasis

Comment   Psoriasis commonly involves penis; penile psoriasis often lacks prominent scale; careful whole-body skin examination is indicated in all patients with genital dermatoses, especially if an STD is not immediately obvious; anxious patients may alter natural appearance of genital lesions by manipulation or self-medication; note similarity to secondary syphilis and scabies (Figs. 4-5, 4-11, 13-2)

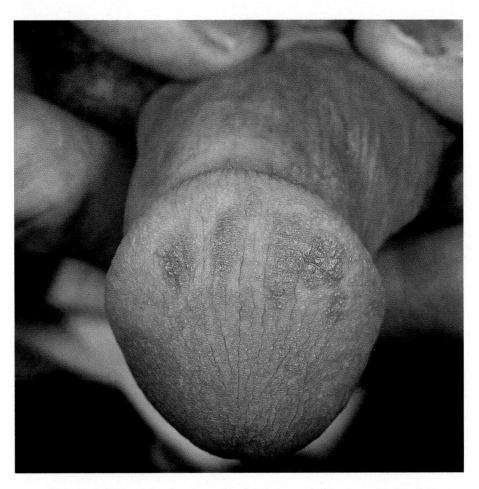

21-4 *Psoriasis. Note absence of prominent scale and similarity to rash of secondary syphilis (Fig. 4-12).*

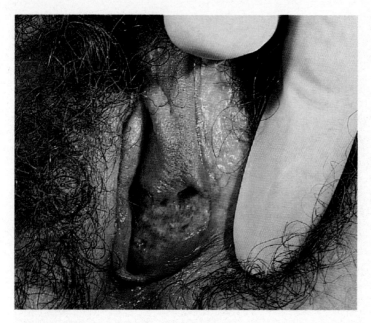

21-5 *Behçet's syndrome.*

Patient Profile Age 23, female married gardener, born in Turkey

History Painful genital sore for 2 weeks; several years of recurrent oral "canker sores"

Examination Large, irregular, deep ulceration of labia; no lymphadenopathy or systemic manifestations; several depressed scars of oral mucosa

Laboratory VDRL, dark-field microscopy, cultures for HSV and *Haemophilus ducreyi* (all negative); biopsy of margin of lesion demonstrated acute inflammation and vasculitis

Diagnosis Behçet's disease

Comment Behçet's disease is a rare and often serious condition manifested by recurrent aggressive oral and genital ulcerations, usually in persons of Mediterranean ancestry; other common manifestations include uveitis, aseptic meningitis, and arteritis involving medium or large arteries; colchicine, glucocorticoids, and cytotoxic drugs are used for treatment, with variable efficacy

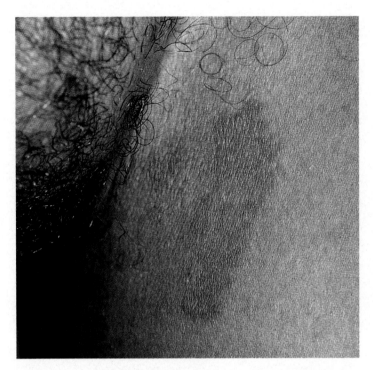

21-6   *Tinea cruris. Caused by dermatophyte fungi (e.g., Trichophyton sp., Epidermophyton sp., Microsporum sp.), tinea cruris ("jock itch") is a common disorder in men but less common in women. It is characterized by erythema of the groin folds and inner thighs, with accentuated erythema and scale at the sharply demarcated advancing border. Tinea pedis (athlete's foot) often is present. The clinical diagnosis usually is reliable, but can be confirmed by scraping the advancing border and examining microscopically for fungal elements after digestion with 10% KOH. Topical imidazole creams (e.g., miconazole) are effective.* (Courtesy of Philip Kirby, M.D.)

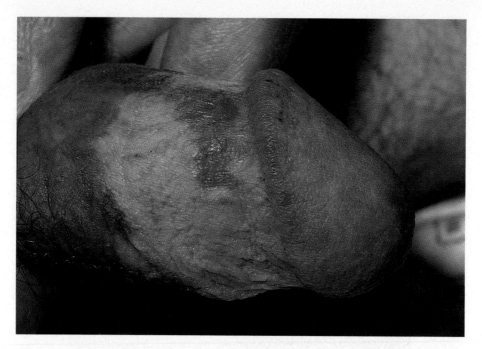

21-7   *Vitiligo of penis. Vitiligo, cutaneous depigmentation of apparent autoimmune etiology, often involves the genitals. It is characterized by sharply demarcated macular areas of total depigmentation; the affected skin is otherwise normal. Vitiligo affects about 1 percent of the population. No reliably effective treatment is known.* (Courtesy of Philip Kirby, M.D.)

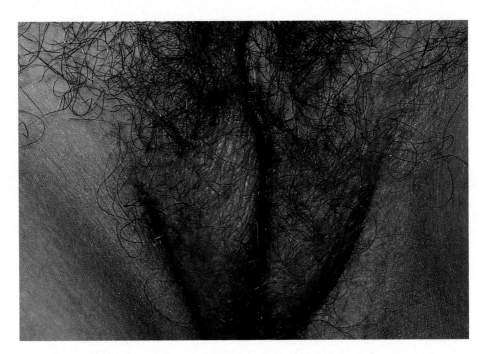

21-8   *Lichen simplex chronicus of the vulva. This disorder usually presents as a solitary, pruritic plaque of thickened, slightly erythematous, scaly skin, with accentuated skin markings (lichenification) and often with overt excoriation. It typically occurs at the base of the scrotum or on the labia majora. The etiology is unknown, but most or all of the clinical findings result directly from repeated scratching and lesions are most common on the side of the patient's dominant hand. Topical steroids and instruction to avoid scratching are usually effective.* (Courtesy of Philip Kirby, M.D.)

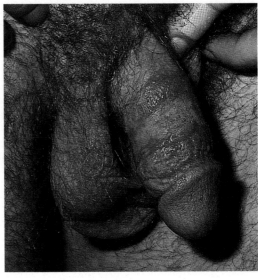

21-9   *Allergic contact dermatitis of penis. This patient was allergic to the adhesive tape of a bandage that he used to cover a recurrence of genital herpes, now healing. Culture of the acutely inflamed lesions was negative for HSV. Allergic contact dermatitis is pruritic and characterized, in its advanced form, by vesicles or a weeping, denuded skin surface. History of exposure to potential irritants or allergens is usually present. Removal of the inciting agent usually is sufficient therapy, although topical steroids may speed resolution.* (Courtesy of Philip Kirby, M.D.)

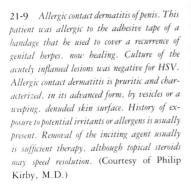

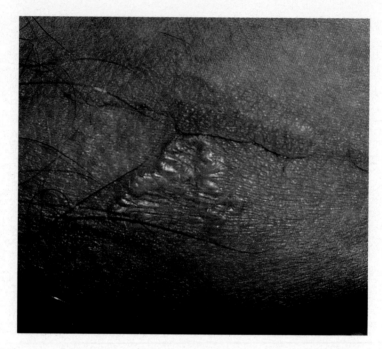

21-10 *Lichen planus of underside of penis. Lichen planus presents with shiny papules and plaques, often annular, with a characteristic lavender or violaceous hue. Nongenital or oral mucosal lesions are often present. Lichen planus can be confused with secondary syphilis. The etiology is unknown. Topical steroids usually are effective.* (Courtesy of Philip Kirby, M.D.)

V   CLINICAL STD SYNDROMES

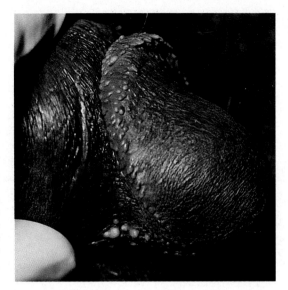

21-11 *Pearly penile papules. Pearly papules are regularly spaced, small (usually 0.5–1.0 mm), shiny papules of the penile corona; prominent papules may have a filiform appearance. This normal anatomic variant is present in up to 10 percent of men, but anxious patients may be concerned (e.g., after observing other men without papules) and naive clinicians may confuse them with warts or other lesions. In this patient, a prominent Tyson's gland (the larger white papule ventrally) is also visible; this also is normal.* (Courtesy of Philip Kirby, M.D.)

ADDITIONAL READING

Fitzpatrick TB et al: *Color Atlas and Synopsis of Clinical Dermatology,* 2d ed. New York, McGraw-Hill, 1992.

Stolz E et al: Other genital dermatoses, in *Sexually Transmitted Diseases,* 2d ed, KK Holmes et al (eds). New York, McGraw-Hill, 1990, chap 60.

Appendix: Medical and Sexual History, Physical Examination, and Laboratory Evaluation of STD Patients

This outline is modified* from the routine screening history, physical examination, and laboratory tests performed on adult and adolescent patients attending the Seattle-King County Department of Public Health STD Clinic at Harborview Medical Center, Seattle. Expanded history, physical examination, or laboratory tests often are required, depending on the initial findings.

MEDICAL HISTORY

Reason for Visit

Symptoms
STD exposure (state STD)
Screening
Other

Symptoms and Duration
MALES

Urethral discharge
Dysuria or urethral pruritus
Genital lesion(s) or rash
Nongenital rash
Anorectal/enteric symptoms
Testicular/scrotal symptoms
Oral/pharyngeal symptoms
Symptoms referable to lymph nodes
Constitutional symptoms
Other symptoms

FEMALES

Abnormal or increased vaginal discharge
Vulvovaginal odor
Dysuria
Urinary frequency or urgency
Genital lesion(s) or rash
Abdominal pain or internal dyspareunia
Nonmenstrual vaginal bleeding
Nongenital rash
Anorectal/enteric symptoms
Oral/pharyngeal symptoms
Symptoms referable to lymph nodes
Constitutional symptoms
Other symptoms

Other Information

Antibiotics in past month (drug, dose, date completed)
Allergies

---

* Clinicians are free to adopt this outline for use in their practices on clinics, without regard to copyright or credit. Most of the elements can be listed in check-off format, with spaces for quantitative information when needed. In the author's STD clinic, all the items for separate male and female charts are included on one side of an 8 × 11.5-in. page, with sufficient space for brief written comments.

Chronic diseases or health problems

Drugs in past year (marijuana, cocaine, narcotics, other)

Alcohol abuse

SEXUAL HISTORY

Sexual Partners

Number of female partners in past 2 and 12 months

Number of male partners in past 2 and 12 months

New partner in past 2 months?

Time since last sexual exposure

Sexual Practices

Sites exposed to partners' genitals or rectum in past 2 months (penis or vagina, rectum, mouth/pharynx)

Condom use with regular partners (always, sometimes, never)

Condom use with casual partners (always, sometimes, never)

Current Contraceptive Method (females only)

Past STD   (lifetime and past 12 months)

Gonorrhea

Chlamydia/NGU/MPC

Herpes

Syphilis

Genital warts/HPV

Trichomoniasis (females)

Bacterial vaginosis (females)

Other

HIV Risk Assessment

Multiple heterosexual partners

Transfusion or blood product therapy, 1977–1985

IV drug use

Acceptance of money or drugs in exchange for sex

Sex since 1977 with:

Homosexual or bisexual men

IV drug users

Prostitutes (male or female)

Sex partner with known or suspected HIV infection

PHYSICAL EXAMINATION

Males

- Inspect penis; retract foreskin; "milk" urethra for discharge by compressing from pubic bone distally to tip of penis
- Palpate scrotal contents
- Inspect anus and perineum if history of rectal sexual exposure; anoscopy if symptoms of proctitis or proctocolitis

Females

- Inspect labia, introitus, meatus, perineum, and anus; palpate abdomen
- Palpate urethra and Bartholin glands
- Speculum examination of vagina and cervix; note amount, character, and site of origin (cervix or vagina) of abnormal exudate
- Anoscopy if symptoms of proctitis or proctocolitis
- Bimanual pelvic examination

Males and Females

- Inspect skin and hair, with emphasis on pubic and inguinal areas, thighs, abdomen, hands, forearms; use bright light; hand magnifier often helpful
- Inspect mouth and throat
- Palpate for cervical, axillary and inguinal lymphadenopahy

ROUTINE LABORATORY TESTS

Males

- For men without symptoms, signs, or epidemiologic suspicion of urethritis, test first 15–20 ml voided urine for pyuria by leukocyte esterase dipstick or microscopy
- If urethritis suspected:

    Gram stain and culture for *N. gonorrhoeae* (external exudate may be used; if none seen, pass urethrogenital swab 2–3 cm into urethra)

    Test for *C. trachomatis* (pass urethrogenital swab 3–4 cm into urethra; external exudate not adequate)

- Rectal and pharyngeal swabs for culture for *N. gonorrhoeae,* if exposed
- Rectal culture for *C. trachomatis,* if exposed (*note:* nonculture tests not recommended for rectal infection)

Females

- Vaginal secretions

    pH (use indicator with pH range 4–7)

    Examine saline preparation microscopically for trichomonads, leukocytes, and clue cells; Gram stain optional (permits assessment of bacterial flora and yeasts but less useful for trichomonads)

    Add 10% KOH and note amine (fishy) odor

    Examine KOH preparation microscopically for yeasts and pseudomycelia (optional if Gram stain shows fungal elements)

- Endocervical tests

    Gram stain (optional when screening asymptomatic women at low risk)

    Culture for *N. gonorrhoeae*

    Test for *C. trachomatis*

Males and Females

- Syphilis serology
- HIV serology and pretest counseling, with consent; if patient declines testing, counsel intensively about sexual safety (as if HIV-positive)
- Hepatitis B serology if high risk

Index

Doxycycline, 12, 25, 34, 63, 127–128, 145, 167, 173
Dysplasia, 5, 85

E

Ectopic pregnancy, 165, 167
ELISA (*see* Enzyme-linked immunosorbent assay)
Enteric infections, 136–137, 172–175
  colitis, 172–173
  enteritis, 172–173
  enterocolitis, 172, 173
  proctocolitis, 172–175, 189
  (*See also* Proctitis)
Enteritis, 172–173
  Campylobacter infection and, 172, 173
  enterocolitis, 172, 173
  epidemiologic history, 172
  epidemiology, 172
  giardiasis, 172–173
  laboratory diagnosis, 173
  physical examination, 173
  salmonellosis and, 172, 173
  sexual orientation, 172
  string test, 173
  symptoms, 172
  transmission, 172
  treatment, 173
Enterocolitis, 172, 173 (*See also* Colitis; Enteritis)
Enzyme immunoassay, 25
Enzyme-linked immunosorbent assay, 98
Epidemiology:
  changes in, 2
  demographic, social, behavioral factors, 2–3
  (*See also specific diseases*)
Epididymitis, 10, 25, 126, 132–135
  age, 132
  causes of, 132
  Chlamydia trachomatis, 132–133
  diagnostic criteria, 133
  epidemiologic history, 132
  epidemiology, 132

Epididymitis (*continued*)
  incidence, 132
  incubation period, 132
  laboratory diagnosis, 132–133
  microbiologic tests, 133
  Neisseria gonorrhoeae, 132–133
  patient profile, 134–135
  physical examination, 132
  prevalence, 132
  Pseudomonas, 132
  sexual orientation, 132
  symptoms, 132
  testicular torsion, 133
  transmission, 132
  treatment, 133
Epstein-Barr virus (EBV), 110
Erythromycin, 12, 25, 34–35, 57, 127–128, 173

F

Fitz-Hugh–Curtis syndrome, 166
Fixed drug eruption, 177
Fluconazole, 155
Fluorescent treponemal antibody-absorbed test, 33
Friability, 144
FTA-ABS (*see* Fluorescent treponemal antibody-absorbed)

G

Ganciclovir, 110
Gardnerella vaginalis, 152
Genital herpes, 68–84, 126
  age, 68
  antiviral chemotherapy, 70
  asymptomatic and subclinical, 69
  clinical classification, 69
  control measures, 71
  core populations for, 3
  counseling, 71
  cytology, 70
  diagnostic criteria, 70
  epidemiologic history, 69